ABC of
# Sleep Medicine

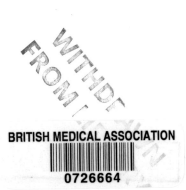

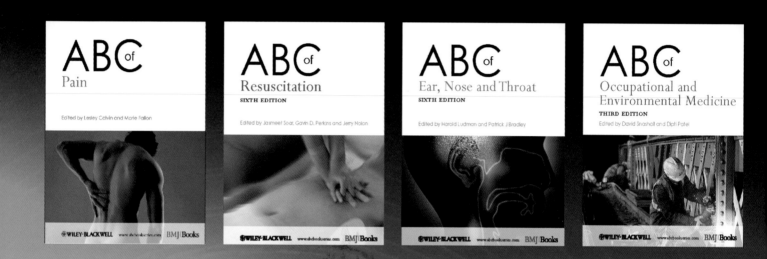

# ABC of

# Sleep Medicine

*Paul Reading*

Consultant Neurologist
Department of Sleep Medicine
James Cook University Hospital
Middlesbrough, UK

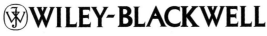

**WILEY-BLACKWELL**
A John Wiley & Sons, Ltd., Publication

**BMJ | Books**

*Library of Congress Cataloging-in-Publication Data*

Reading, Paul.
  ABC of sleep medicine / Paul Reading.
       p. ; cm.
  Includes bibliographical references and index.
  ISBN 978-0-470-65946-5 (pbk.)
  I. Title.
  [DNLM: 1. Sleep Disorders–pathology. 2. Sleep–physiology. WL 108]
  616.8′498–dc23
                                              2012035462

A catalogue record for this book is available from the British Library.

Wiley also publishes its books in a variety of electronic formats. Some content that appears in print may not be available in electronic books.

Cover design by: Meaden Creative

Set in 9.25/12 Minion by Laserwords Private Limited, Chennai, India
Printed and bound in Malaysia by Vivar Printing Sdn Bhd

1   2013

# Contents

# Preface

At a personal level, everyone recognises the importance of good quality sleep. From a medical perspective, however, only recently has the potential adverse impact of a disordered sleep–wake cycle on cognitive, mental and even physical health been realised. The consequences of excessive daytime sleepiness are also increasingly defined, especially with respect to driving and other potentially dangerous activities. Perhaps surprisingly, the precise biological reasons why every animal has a basic need for regular sleep are still speculative and the fascinating state of rapid eye movement (REM) sleep remains a particular enigma. However, it is abundantly clear that sleepiness is a true drive state and, ultimately, as important as hunger or thirst for optimal health and survival.

Partly because it cuts across numerous more established specialities, the emerging discipline of sleep medicine remains in its infancy and is generally poorly addressed in medical schools. As a consequence, many physicians in primary and secondary care lack confidence in addressing sleep-related symptoms, despite significant advances in our understanding and treatment options for the majority of sleep disorders over the last decade. A further confound is a widely held and mistaken belief that sleep disorders invariably require complex and expensive techniques for confident diagnosis. With the exception of sleep-related breathing disorders, the majority of sleep disorders can actually be adequately managed without an absolute need for detailed investigations.

This book has been written as a primer for understanding the fascinating phenomenon of sleep and its commoner disorders. The aim has been to provide a readable text for non-specialists, covering the full range of recognised sleep disorders that might present to general physicians and sleep clinics. Throughout, it is emphasised that a full sleep–wake history, potentially corroborated by close family members, together with a basic knowledge of sleep neurobiology, will usually allow an accurate diagnosis and potential treatment options. The full range of diagnostic sleep investigations is also discussed in some detail, outlining when they are appropriate but also highlighting pitfalls in interpretation. Of course, it is often difficult to know whether sleep-related symptoms reflect a defined disorder or simply result from social or psychological factors; grey areas undoubtedly remain. However, symptomatic 'red flags' are highlighted which may indicate the need for more specialist attention.

A particularly difficult area in sleep medicine is the scarcity of a controlled evidence base to guide treatment protocols. As an inevitable consequence, the reader should be aware that many suggestions for medications mentioned in this text are personal recommendations, based largely on anecdotal evidence. Furthermore, it should be noted that it is rare for a drug to have a formal licence for use in sleep medicine.

Sleep clinics, at least in the United Kingdom, are increasing in numbers but remain variable in their ability to address the whole gamut of sleep disorders. The majority are primarily concerned with managing the important condition of obstructive sleep apnoea but lack expertise in neurological or psychological aspects of sleep disorders. A working knowledge of the whole spectrum of sleep disorders is therefore essential for primary care physicians, especially since symptoms of impaired sleep or reduced daytime alertness are amongst the commonest complaints. Not infrequently, a potentially disabling and treatable condition such as narcolepsy may be missed if an incomplete history is elicited. This book will hopefully introduce non-specialists to sleep medicine and increase confidence in how to approach sleep-related symptoms, removing some of the mystique surrounding this fascinating and important area of medicine.

Paul Reading

# CHAPTER 1

# Normal versus Abnormal Sleep

## OVERVIEW

- Sleep almost certainly serves a vital function at the cellular level and is an absolute requirement for every animal
- In large population studies across the globe, chronically poor or insufficient sleep appears to correlate with increased mortality, arterial disease, diabetes and possibly cancer rates
- Sleep is highly orchestrated into discrete cycles of non-rapid eye movement (non-REM) and rapid eye movement (REM) stages
- Vivid dreams most often occur from the REM sleep stage
- Increasing age dramatically alters sleep quality and consolidation
- If insufficient deep non-REM sleep is obtained during a night, subjects will generally awake unrefreshed
- REM sleep is a very active brain state which has been proposed to facilitate memory consolidation and emotional processing although its true function ultimately remains obscure
- At least 90% of the adult population benefit from 7–8 hours of good sleep per night
- Around 5% of the population can be considered excessively sleepy during the day although increased sleepiness may not be recognised as such and may be expressed through other symptoms
- During nocturnal sleep, a variety of bodily movements is experienced normally

## The importance of sleep

Virtually everyone acknowledges that significantly disturbed sleep has profound and immediate adverse effects on mental, cognitive and even physical well-being. However, the true long-term importance of good sleep for optimal general health may not yet be fully recognised.

The fact that every animal has evolved to have an absolute need for regular sleep in order to survive clearly suggests that it performs some vital and, as yet, ill-defined function. Intuitively, sleep appears to facilitate restoration and repair. Almost certainly, however, it has much more than a simple passive or restful role. In many respects, sleep is an active brain state and is not merely the

absence of wakefulness. Indeed, during rapid eye movement (REM) sleep, the brain is as metabolically active as during wakefulness. As a consequence, some authorities have termed REM sleep as 'paradoxical sleep'.

In recent animal models, it appears that being awake for just a few hours vigorously activates metabolic 'cell stress' or adaptive biochemical pathways. This response to prolonged wakefulness is seen particularly in nerve cells that appear to be protecting themselves from damage and potential early death or apoptosis. It is therefore conceivable that any excess of wakefulness is the potentially damaging factor rather than a lack of sleep *per se*.

It is clearly difficult to study the long-term consequences of bad sleep in humans. Of interest, however, a large prospective four-year study of healthy elderly subjects suggested that the only reliable predictor of death or subsequent dependency from a large number of demographic details was a complaint of disordered sleep, particularly in males.

A renowned sleep researcher (William Dement) famously stated that 'Sleep is of the brain, for the brain and by the brain', emphasising the adverse effects of poor sleep predominantly on brain function and mental health. Conversely, virtually every central nervous system and mental health disorder has the potential to disturb the sleep–wake cycle. Furthermore, chronic poor quality or insufficient sleep may actively fuel many common conditions, such as generalised pain syndromes and affective disorders. This strongly suggests that sleep has a 'bi-directional' relationship with many common conditions (Figure 1.1).

In many situations, it is possible that direct attention both to sleep quantity and quality may have indirect and positive effects on an unexpected range of health issues. In this respect, the established epidemiological links between chronic sleep deprivation (less than six hours a night) and diabetes, hypertension, vascular disease or even cancer are increasingly germane. The difficult and important question of whether increasing quantity or quality of sleep in 'at risk' populations will positively affect outcome remains to be established.

## Defining sleep

The loose behavioural definition of sleep as a temporary and reversible state of altered consciousness and perceptual disengagement has been superseded by electrophysiological criteria.

*ABC of Sleep Medicine*, First Edition. Paul Reading.
© 2013 John Wiley & Sons, Ltd. Published 2013 by John Wiley & Sons, Ltd.

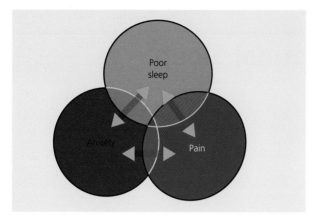

**Figure 1.1** Chronically poor quality or insufficient sleep is rarely an isolated problem. For example, pain and anxiety may well impede good sleep but sleep restriction or impairment can also increase sensitivity to pain and raise anxiety levels.

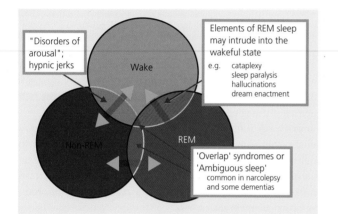

**Figure 1.2** The brain can be considered as normally existing in the three mutually exclusive states of WAKE, non-REM or REM sleep. Orchestrated transitions between these states occur automatically and relatively quickly over the 24-hour period. In many sleep disorders, particularly the parasomnias, the switch between states may be inefficient or incomplete.

Although simplistic, it is valid to consider three distinct and mutually exclusive brain states, namely wakefulness, rapid eye movement (REM) sleep and non-REM sleep (Figure 1.2). Switches between these states should occur automatically, quickly and relatively seamlessly. A large proportion of sleep disorders is associated with inefficient, faulty or incomplete states of transition.

Non-REM sleep can be divided into light (stages 1 and 2) or deep phases (stages 3 and 4) on the basis of the surface cerebral electroencephalogram (EEG) (Figure 1.3). Around 20% of the night is spent in the curious state of REM sleep, in which most of the cerebral cortex and limbic system is extremely active, as confirmed by recent functional brain imaging studies. In contrast to this enhanced metabolic activity, there are descending inhibitory neural impulses from the brainstem that innervate the vast majority of peripheral muscles during REM sleep, rendering the subject floppy (atonic) and areflexic.

REM sleep loosely correlates with the normal phenomena of dreams or nightmares, usually recalled briefly if a subject is awoken

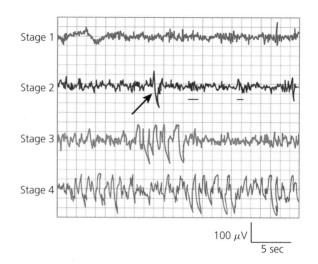

**Figure 1.3** Representative electroencephalographic (EEG) traces of the 4 stages of non-REM sleep. The arrow indicates a K-complex, one of the hallmarks of light non-REM sleep. Large amplitude delta (slow) waves dominate the trace in deep non-REM sleep (stages 3 and 4).
In recently revised criteria for sleep staging, light non-REM sleep (stages 1 and 2) has been designated as N1 whereas deep non-REM (stages 3 and 4) is N2. This revision has not been completely accepted internationally at the time of writing.

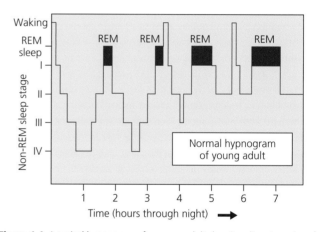

**Figure 1.4** A typical hypnogram of a young adult showing discrete cycles of non-REM and REM sleep through the night. Deep non-REM sleep predominates in the first third whereas REM sleep is most dense in the last third. Brief awakenings are often not recognised. If they occur during REM sleep, a vivid dream would be expected.

from this stage of sleep. However, less vivid or bizarre 'sleep mentation', usually without a narrative thread, is also frequently reported if arousals from sleep occur from non-REM sleep stages.

An ideal nocturnal sleep in young adults consists of four or five cycles of REM/non-REM sleep with deep non-REM sleep dominating the first third of the night and REM sleep the last third (Figure 1.4). Minor arousals from sleep are common, especially with increasing age, and often not registered or recalled.

## How much sleep is needed?

There is clearly a degree of individual variation in the optimum length of the nocturnal sleep period but probably 90% of adults

**Table 1.1** A selected list of the neuropsychological effects secondary to acute sleep deprivation.

| Main neuropsychological effect of acute sleep deprivation | Year of study |
| --- | --- |
| Increased reaction times | 1988 |
| Perseveration and reduced flexibility | 1999 |
| Impaired sense of humour | 2006 |
| Increased risk taking | 2007 |
| Impaired moral judgement | 2007 |
| Reduced emotional intelligence | 2010 |
| Increased 'negativity' with enhanced memory for adverse events | 2010 |
| Increased distractibility | 2010 |

require at least seven hours of good quality sleep. For most people, sleeping regularly for six hours or less produces objective signs of reduced vigilance, even if subjective sleepiness is minimal.

Although sleepiness is the obvious consequence of acute sleep deprivation, increasingly, a number of studies have demonstrated neuropsychological effects (Table 1.1). The majority of these can be interpreted in terms of temporary frontal lobe dysfunction. Many have commented that the sleep-deprived brain of a young adult functions in a similar way to the brain in extreme old age.

Although underlying mechanisms are unclear and precise interpretation is difficult, several enormous population studies have consistently reported increased mortality, vascular disease and diabetes in those reporting less than five hours of sleep per night when followed up for several years. Intriguingly, those sleeping for more than 9.5 hours a night similarly have reduced longevity.

Increasingly, it is realised that the nature of sleep may be as crucially important as its quantity, although precise definitions of sleep quality are poorly defined. The absolute amount of deep non-REM (slow wave) sleep through the night may predict how refreshed a subject feels in the morning but other measures, such as the time spent awake after sleep onset, may also be used as surrogate markers of quality.

The true function of REM sleep remains a mystery. Most awakenings from REM sleep are associated with vivid dreams that often have a bizarre narrative, incorporating elements of recent events or more distant memories. Psychoanalytic explanations of dreams in terms of 'wish fulfilment' have largely been superseded by more biological explanations. However, it remains unclear whether it is the dream itself or the underlying neurobiological processes behind REM sleep that are more important.

A common thread with much recent research on REM sleep function concerns memory processing or consolidation. In brief, one influential view is that the brain restructures or consolidates certain forms of memory through a form of rehearsal when 'off-line' during REM sleep. It is likely that processing of emotional memories is a particularly important function. Many cognitive tasks seem to improve after a period of sleep and some evidence even supports the notion that unexpected insights into mathematical problems occur during the unconscious state of sleep.

The study of dreams, oneirology, has a rich history. Many theories regarding dream function and REM sleep have been generated. Some interesting facts concerning REM sleep are listed in Box 1.1.

> **Box 1.1  Interesting facts about REM or 'paradoxical' sleep**
>
> - Almost one third of the first few months of life are spent in a form of REM sleep.
> - In animal experiments, preventing rats from entering REM sleep for around four weeks has fatal consequences.
> - There are profound autonomic changes during REM sleep causing 'instability' of pulse rate and blood pressure. In theory, this might predispose certain individuals to cardiac arrhythmias during REM sleep.
> - Thermoregulation is absent during REM sleep. If the environment is too hot or cold, arousals from sleep are particularly likely during the REM stage.
> - Many drugs, including alcohol, suppress REM sleep. If stopped abruptly after prolonged intake, such drugs lead to rebound symptoms, including vivid dreaming or even visual hallucinations.
> - Depressed patients enter REM sleep more quickly.
> - The majority of antidepressant drugs suppress or delay REM sleep.
> - Domestic animals have significantly more REM sleep than their feral counterparts.

It is often overlooked that sleepiness, like thirst or hunger, is a true drive state which builds up during prolonged wakefulness and will only be satiated by sleep itself. The neurobiological substrates of sleepiness and the underlying homeostatic mechanisms remain poorly understood although accumulation of the neurochemical adenosine in certain key areas, such as the basal forebrain, may be crucial. Indeed, caffeine works to offset the sleep drive by inhibiting adenosine receptors in these areas.

Superimposed on the homeostatic sleep drive are circadian factors which confer additional levels of somnolence at certain times of the day, irrespective of the immediate sleep history. These 'dips' in alertness, seen particularly at 3.00 p.m. and 4.00 a.m., may have consequences for behaviour and explain the rise in sleep-related traffic accidents at these times.

The fascinating field of chronobiology has provided a sound scientific basis for understanding the mechanisms of our internal clocks. Remarkably, the molecular machinery at a subcellular level has been largely established and hardly differs across all species studied from fruit flies to humans. The suprachiasmatic nucleus, a small area in the hypothalamus comprising around 25 000 neurons, has been established as the 'master clock', with the capacity to influence all circadian rhythms throughout the body (Figure 1.5).

## The effects of age

The quantity and, particularly, the quality of sleep change enormously across the normal lifespan. Newborns typically spend over half of the 24-hour period in a state resembling REM sleep. They have wakeful episodes lasting two or three hours interspersed with similar relatively short sleep periods across the day–night period. In the first two years, a prolonged nocturnal sleep usually

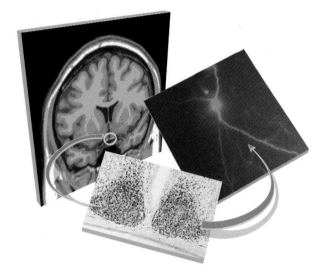

**Figure 1.5** The suprachiasmatic nucleus in the hypothalamus is circled with magnification of the cellular component. This small area of the brain contains around 25 000 neurons but is the 'master' timekeeper of all circadian rhythms in the body.

**Table 1.2** Questions for assessing increased somnolence.

| Question or probe | Implications for positive answer |
| --- | --- |
| Are you waking up from naps without realising you had been sleep? | Indicates 'sleep attacks'; can be seen in any cause of severe excessive sleepiness such as narcolepsy |
| Given the chance, could you nap more than once a day? | Implies excessive sleepiness rather than, for example, simple fatigue |
| Have you fallen asleep in unusual situations, such as in public (e.g. on buses, in shops)? | Implies significantly excessive sleepiness |
| Do you regularly fall asleep within a few minutes when a passenger in a car? | May indicate significant sleepiness |
| Do you routinely fall asleep when watching films on television? | May indicate significant sleepiness |
| Have friends or family commented on you dropping off to sleep inappropriately? | Usually implies excessive sleepiness, particularly in some situations where it may not be appreciated by the subject (e.g. Parkinson's disease or dementia) |
| Are you prone to frequent lapses or 'automatic' behaviours (e.g. placing objects in inappropriate places or losing items around the house)? | May imply 'microsleeps' or brief periods of inattention as an indication of significant sleepiness |
| At times do you find it very hard to concentrate or take in new information? | Particularly in those who fight the urge to sleep, it might not be appreciated that impaired vigilance and concentration are early markers of significant sleepiness |
| Do you feel hyperactive at times and unable to focus or attend to a simple task? | Distractibility resembling attention deficit and hyperactivity disorder (ADHD) may reflect underlying sleepiness, particularly in children |

becomes established, invariably encouraged by parental input, with afternoon naps remaining the norm until around five years of age.

The commonest pattern through teenage life is for sleep onset to become progressively later. Although lifestyle factors and habits may fuel this tendency, there is also evidence that most teenagers have internal clock mechanisms predisposing them to become 'night owls'. The most obvious practical consequence of this pattern is extreme difficulty arising at a conventional hour for educational purposes.

Beyond adolescence, however, the brain's internal clock tends to 'advance'. With each subsequent decade, the natural desire to sleep typically occurs around 30 minutes earlier.

The most striking age-related change in sleep patterns relates to a progressive deterioration in sleep consolidation. Several minor arousals, usually later in the night, might be considered normal in early middle-age. In the healthy elderly, frank sleep fragmentation is extremely common. The depth of slow wave sleep (non-REM stages 3 and 4) also reduces dramatically with age, with the earliest changes evident in males as young as 25.

The increased depth of non-REM sleep in younger subjects accounts for the extreme difficulty often encountered if children need to be woken from deep sleep in the first third of the night. Forced arousals frequently produce apparent confusion or 'sleep drunkenness', a phenomenon also frequently observed in sleep-deprived adults.

## When is daytime sleepiness abnormal?

Although napping most afternoons is clearly a normal phenomenon, in many Mediterranean cultures, for example, the propensity to fall asleep through the day if rested or unoccupied may well indicate an underlying disorder. Increased somnolence is usually different to simple tiredness or fatigue and particular care is needed in nomenclature and obtaining an accurate history. Some useful leading questions are given in Table 1.2.

Probably 5% of the population can be considered to have excessive daytime somnolence that potentially interferes with daily activities. The dangers of impaired wakefulness or alertness when engaged in tasks such as driving or operating machinery are obvious.

One of the first signs of excessive sleepiness is the presence of minor lapses or 'microsleeps'. These last up to three seconds, during which time there is incomplete awareness or attention to events in the external world. A further consequence of reduced alertness is impaired cognitive processing, particularly in tasks requiring vigilance and short-term memory. Indeed, it is not uncommon for severe hypersomnolence to masquerade clinically as a dementing illness.

With increasing levels of daytime somnolence, subjects are prone to automatic behaviours, performing tasks on 'auto pilot' with no clear subsequent recollection. Typically, objects are either lost around the house or placed in inappropriate locations. A common situation in severe sleepiness is for the subject to carrying on writing or texting whilst half asleep, producing nonsense prose or unintelligible handwriting.

## Normal nocturnal motor phenomena during sleep

It is normal to exhibit some movement even during deep sleep. Involuntary simple shifts of body position every 20 minutes or so reflect the commonest phenomenon. However, vigorous so-called hypnic jerks at the point of sleep onset are also common, particularly in young or sleep deprived subjects. Occasionally, such jerks occur in association with alarming sensory symptoms, such as 'flashes' or 'bangs'. The extreme variety of this generally benign phenomenon has been called 'exploding head syndrome' and can be a potent cause for sleep-onset insomnia.

During REM sleep, all voluntary movements except those involving the diaphragm and oculomotor muscles are actively inhibited by descending pathways from the brainstem to the motor neurones. However, minor intermittent (myoclonic) jerks of limbs or facial muscles are frequently seen. Arousals to full wakefulness from REM sleep are also very common, especially late in the night, usually in association with vivid dreams or even disturbing nightmares.

Leg movements resembling a slow withdrawal reflex may recur in bursts every 20 seconds or so during all stages of sleep. Such periodic limb movements (PLMs) may be observed in up to a third of the normal elderly population and are most often a benign epiphenomenon. However, if PLMs are particularly violent or observed in association with significant restless legs syndrome, sleep may be disturbed. Drug therapy may be warranted, if only to improve the sleep quality of the bed partner.

## Conclusions

At a personal level, everyone appreciates how important good sleep is for optimum health and vitality. However, determining when a reportedly disturbed sleep–wake cycle reflects a defined sleep disorder can be difficult, since many of the associated symptoms form part of a normal spectrum. However, chronically poor sleep, particularly in association with the inevitable adverse effects of natural ageing, may actively fuel many common complaints, such as headaches, generalised pain and depressed mood.

Sleep is also an important and often overlooked consideration in the majority of general medical conditions. Because sleep medicine is a young and poorly defined discipline in most countries, education given to medical students is generally limited. As a likely consequence, the quality of clinical practice varies enormously. The increasingly recognised relevance of sleep medicine to public health will hopefully improve future resources.

Treatments for the whole spectrum of sleep disorders are established and are becoming both evidence based and increasingly sophisticated. A common dilemma in general practice is when to refer to a sleep centre for specialist advice. Severity of symptoms is often a sufficient prompt. However, Table 1.3 provides a selection of 'red flags' which, if they accompany a sleep-related symptom, might merit referral for further assessment and possible investigation.

We are still some way from understanding the true function of sleep but the adverse consequences of its dysfunction are becoming clearer across all areas of general medicine and psychiatry.

**Table 1.3** 'Red flags' which might merit referral for further assessment.

| Sleep-related symptom | Selected 'red flags' from history that might indicate need for further specialist assessment |
| --- | --- |
| Excessive daytime sleepiness (not simple tiredness or fatigue) | Feeling the need to sleep in potentially dangerous situations, such as behind the steering wheel<br>Sudden episodes of sleep with little or no warning of the imperative to sleep ('sleep attacks')<br>Historical evidence for overnight sleep apnoea or waking unrefreshed with severe dryness of mouth<br>Other symptoms, such as cataplexy, that suggest a primary (central) sleep disorder |
| Sleep-onset insomnia | Evidence for significant restless legs syndrome before sleep interfering with sleep onset<br>Inability to rise at a conventional hour might suggest a 'clock' problem, such as delayed sleep phase syndrome |
| Sleep-maintenance insomnia | If there is accompanying frank daytime sleepiness, it is likely there is a defined medical reason for poor quality sleep<br>The younger the patient, the more likely there is a defined cause for interrupted overnight sleep |
| Nocturnal motor activity suggesting a parasomnia | Potentially dangerous or frequent behaviours<br>Accompanying significant daytime sleepiness might indicate presence of another sleep disorder fuelling parasomnia |
| | New onset of parasomnia activity is unusual beyond 40 years of age and might suggest REM sleep abnormalities associated with other disorders such as Parkinson's disease |
| | Features that might suggest an epileptic cause for nocturnal motor activity (Chapter 7) |

## Further reading

Altena. E, Ramautar, J.R., Van der Werf, Y.D. and Van Someren, E.J. (2010) Do sleep complaints contribute to age-related cognitive decline? *Prog Brain Res*, **185**, 181–205.

Axelsson, J., Sundelin, T., Ingre, M. *et al.* (2010) Beauty sleep: experimental study on the perceived health and attractiveness of sleep deprived people. *BMJ*, **341**, c6614

Cappuccio, F.P., D'Elia, L., Strazzullo, P. and Miller, M.A. (2010) Sleep duration and all-cause mortality: a systematic review and meta-analysis of prospective studies. *Sleep* , **33**, 582–595.

Frank, M.G. (2006) The mystery of sleep function: current perspectives and future directions. *Rev Neurosciences*, **17**, 375–392.

Knutson, K.L., Spiegel, K., Penev, P. and van Cauter, E. (2007) The metabolic consequences of sleep deprivation. *Sleep Med*, **11**, 163–178.

Pollak, C.P., Derlick, P., Linsner, J.P., Wenston, J. and Hsieh F. (1990) Sleep problems in the community elderly as predictors of death and nursing home placement. *J Community Health*, **15**, 123–135.

Reynolds, A.C. and Banks, S. (2010) Total sleep deprivation, chronic sleep restriction and sleep disruption. *Prog Brain Res*, **185**, 91–103.

# CHAPTER 2

# Diagnosing Sleep Disorders

### OVERVIEW

- If available, a reliable sleep history is generally more useful than sleep investigations in diagnosing sleep disorders
- Cyclical dips in blood oxygen saturations overnight form the basis of diagnosing sleep apnoea syndromes and can be demonstrated by simple home oximetry tests in most cases
- Sophisticated home ambulatory recording equipment can be used to confirm sleep apnoea if there is diagnostic doubt
- Full overnight polysomnography provides a clear objective snapshot of a subject's sleep quality but always needs to be analysed in a clinical or symptom-based context
- Accurately measuring objective levels of sleepiness and wakefulness is very difficult, partly due to uncertainties over the normal range
- The multiple sleep latency test (MSLT) and maintenance of wakefulness test (MWT) are considered 'gold standards' for measuring or quantifying levels of sleepiness but are very sensitive to procedural variations and protocols
- Actigraphy is a simple technique that gives a useful approximation of a subject's sleep–wake cycle over a period of weeks by continuously measuring limb movements

Box 2.1 **The eight main categories of sleep disorder as defined by the International Classification of Sleep Disorders (ICSD) manual (2nd edition)**

1 Insomnia
2 Sleep-related breathing disorders
3 Hypersomnias of central origin, not due to breathing disorders or other causes of disturbed sleep
4 Circadian rhythm sleep disorders
5 Parasomnias
6 Sleep-related movement disorders
7 Isolated symptoms, possible normal variants and unresolved issues
8 Other sleep disorders

Largely due to the perceived mysterious nature of sleep and the difficulties in investigating it, many clinicians lack confidence when diagnosing sleep disorders. This partly reflects the wide spectrum between normal and abnormal but also reflects the relatively low profile of sleep medicine in most educational curricula.

The most widely accepted international classification of sleep disorders (ICSD) was last revised in 2005 and outlines eight major categories (Box 2.1). Although a useful and exhaustive guide, it is written from a largely American perspective that it not always applicable or appropriate to clinical practice in other countries. Furthermore, it is clear that the relatively new field of sleep medicine continues to evolve rapidly and that many uncertainties and ambiguities remain.

A common misperception amongst non-specialists is that sophisticated investigative techniques are invariably needed for accurately diagnosing sleep disorders. However, a directed and reliable sleep history is almost invariably more useful than sleep tests (Table 2.1). Clearly, difficulties may arise if helpful or essential collaborative information from a bed partner or family member is not available. A self-completed sleep diary for at least two weeks can be a useful addition to history taking (Figure 5.2 shows an example).

This chapter will focus on diagnostic investigations used to confirm clinically suspected sleep disorders. It should be emphasised that information from sleep testing is not always diagnostic in itself and invariably needs to be taken in context with a patient's sleep–wake symptoms of concern. It is not rare for minor abnormalities picked up on sleep tests to be misleading or misinterpreted.

## Tests for sleep-related breathing disorders

Before embarking on formal treatment for a sleep-related breathing disorder such as obstructive sleep apnoea (OSA), it is mandatory to provide some objective evidence to confirm the diagnosis.

Many clinics specialising in sleep apnoea will only accept patients for a diagnostic work-up if there are associated indications of daytime hypersomnolence. The most commonly accepted simple screen for assessing levels of somnolence is the Epworth scale. In this subjective assessment, a subject has to rate the chances of falling asleep (between 0 and 3) over the previous few weeks in eight routine situations (Box 2.2). A score of over 10/24 on the scale

*ABC of Sleep Medicine*, First Edition. Paul Reading.
© 2013 John Wiley & Sons, Ltd. Published 2013 by John Wiley & Sons, Ltd.

**Table 2.1** Some important sleep-related symptoms and their implications.

| Sleep-related symptom | Implications |
|---|---|
| Short sleep time (<6 hours) | Short sleeper (constitutional); all types of insomnia; consider depression; circadian rhythm disorder (especially delayed sleep phase syndrome [DSPS]) |
| Irregular sleep times | Social or work related; circadian rhythm disorder |
| Delay in falling asleep | Sleep-onset insomnia, look for secondary cause(s) |
| Difficulty waking in morning | Sleep deprivation; sleep inertia (sleep 'drunkenness'); idiopathic hypersomnolence |
| Restless during night | Frequent arousals (look for causes of secondary sleep-maintenance insomnia); obstructive sleep apnoea; periodic limb movements during sleep; rarely epileptic phenomena |
| Complex movements during sleep | Parasomnias; nocturnal epilepsy may need to be considered |
| Snoring | Simple or primary snoring with no adverse consequences to the subject; upper airway resistance syndrome; obstructive sleep apnoea |
| Nocturnal choking | Obstructive sleep apnoea; gastro-oesophageal reflux; vocal cord adduction causing stridor; panic attacks |
| Unrefreshing sleep | Sleep restriction; all causes of secondary sleep-maintenance insomnia, including conditions associated with hyper-arousal such as fibromyalgia |
| Daily early morning headache | Carbon dioxide retention; obstructive sleep apnoea |
| Daytime naps | Insufficient sleep; all causes of secondary insomnia; narcolepsy; idiopathic hypersomnia |
| Weakness, localised or general, with emotion | Cataplexy, invariably in association with narcolepsy |
| Pre-sleep apprehension | Anxiety; psychophysiological insomnia; fear of event during sleep (nightmares, parasomnias) |
| Pre-sleep leg discomfort and movements | Restless legs syndrome and associated periodic limb movements |

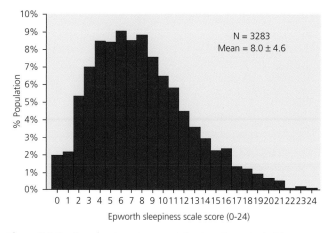

**Figure 2.1** Daytime sleepiness in a population-based sample. In this representative sample of the general population, almost 20% scored 11 or over on the Epworth scale, indicating possible excessive daytime sleepiness. Severe OSA patients or those with narcolepsy would be expected to score 15 or over.

is often taken as the arbitrary criterion for accepting referrals to a sleep apnoea clinic.

The Epworth scale is easy to administer but highly subjective, with a significant range of normality in the general population (Figure 2.1). Furthermore, some of the questions may not be valid or appropriate for certain individuals, including children.

## Oximetry

Ambulatory oximetry is a simple and inexpensive screening tool for OSA that can be undertaken in a subject's home. A finger probe measures oxyhaemoglobin saturation during the recording period of one or more nights along with pulse rate (Figure 2.2). In clear cut cases of sleep apnoea, a characteristic pattern of saturation dips with associated pulse rises is seen (Figure 2.3a and 2.3b). A desaturation index of significant oxygen dips per hour measuring more than 4% is often taken as a useful guide of OSA severity.

---

Box 2.2 **The eight stem situations from the Epworth scale in which a subject is asked to assess their propensity to sleep**

- Sitting and reading
- Watching TV
- Sitting inactive in a public place (e.g. theatre or meeting)
- Sitting as a passenger in a car for an hour without a break
- Lying down to rest in the afternoon when circumstances permit
- Sitting and talking to someone
- Sitting quietly after lunch without alcohol
- Sitting in a car while stopped for a few minutes in traffic

Patient rates each item as    0 (would never doze) to
    3 (high chance of dozing)

ESS total score:    0 → 24

ESS = Epworth sleep scale

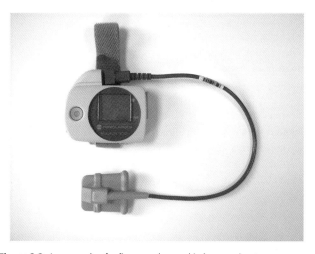

**Figure 2.2** An example of a finger probe used in home oximetry.

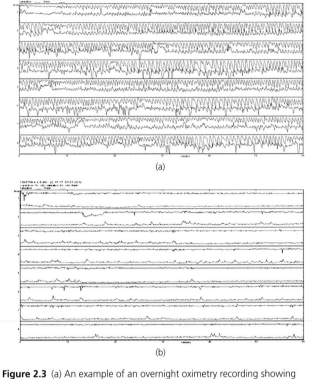

**Figure 2.3** (a) An example of an overnight oximetry recording showing numerous cyclical dips in oxygen concentration through the night (red lines) and significant pulse rate variability (blue lines); this indicates severe sleep apnoea. (b) A normal overnight oximeter recording for comparison.

**Table 2.2** Factors influencing the diagnostic yield of ambulatory oximetry in OSA.

| Patient factors | Body habitus | Obese subjects have decreased functional residual capacity with reduced oxygen stores; relative hypoxaemia may produce false positive data |
|---|---|---|
| | Underlying pulmonary disease | Persistently low oxygen saturations may produce false positive results because the oxyhaemoglobin dissociation curve is steep |
| | Patient sleep status | Oximetry does not detect sleep; if awake, false negative data may be obtained |
| Technical factors | Positioning of probe | Artefact is common due to incorrect positioning or factors such as nail varnish, thick or pigmented skin |
| | Sampling rates | The oximeter can be programmed to have different 'response times' which can give major variations in output data |
| Defining abnormal results | Studies have differing criteria for abnormal levels of apnoeas and hypopnoeas | Oxygen desaturation index may be better guide; small oscillations in desaturation levels may be difficult to interpret |

Published data imply considerable range in both the specificity (40–100%) and sensitivity (25–99%) of oximetry, reflecting the many factors that may influence the quality or reliability of the test (Table 2.2). If there is strong clinical suspicion and inconclusive data from simple oximetry, more sophisticated testing is usually appropriate.

Oximetry is commonly used to confirm treatment outcomes for sleep apnoea at clinical follow-up.

## Home ambulatory recordings with movement detectors and respiratory monitors

Increasingly, more sophisticated home recordings are undertaken, particularly if there remains diagnostic doubt after simple oximetry.

One widely available type of equipment uses additional chest muscle leads to record respiratory effort and electromyographic electrodes on limbs to monitor gross movements. Along with oxygen desaturation patterns and pulse rate changes, the additional data may confirm OSA and help to exclude central sleep apnoea (Chapter 4) as a cause for dips in oxygen saturation. If excessive limb movements are recorded at regular intervals, periodic limb movement disorder (PLMD) may be considered in the differential diagnosis.

## Polysomnography

There is little doubt that full polysomnography (PSG) remains the 'gold standard' investigation for sleep physicians. By measuring multiple parameters simultaneously it allows sleep to be accurately staged and its overall quality assessed with respect to variables such as limb movements and breathing. However, it is expensive, requires the input of skilled technologists and usually requires the subject to sleep in an unfamiliar environment whilst heavily monitored. The availability and, most likely, the quality of PSG vary greatly from region to region.

A typical PSG set-up will have at least the following features:

- Two electrodes placed centrally near the vertex to record the surface electroencephalogram (EEG), vital in sleep staging;
- Electrodes around each eye to monitor movements of the globe, especially to record REM sleep;
- Electromyographic electrodes under the chin and on each shin to measure muscle movement and tone, essential for recording the usual lack of muscle tone in REM sleep and for measuring periodic limb movements;
- Oximetry recording;
- Chest and abdominal leads to record 'strain' and muscular effort during respiration;
- An accelerometer to record body position and shifting of position;
- Audio and video recording under low level or infrared lighting;
- Electrocardiographic (ECG) monitoring.

Optional additional EEG electrodes (up to 12) may be placed over the skull if epileptic seizures are in the differential diagnosis. Nasal and mouth airflow can be assessed indirectly by thermistors

## Summary Graph

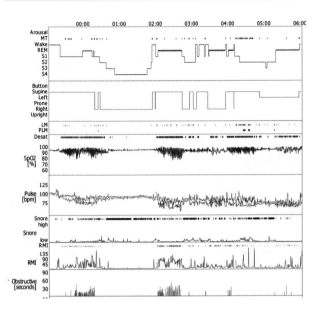

**Figure 2.4** Overall, the trace reveals severe sleep apnoea that is primarily obstructive in nature, worse when the subject is lying supine and with some relation to REM sleep. Sleep is generally fragmented and numerous leg movements are seen, mostly in relation to respiratory events.

that record temperature changes between inspired and expired air. In some specialised units, a small oesophageal balloon can be introduced to record intra-thoracic pressure as an accurate index of respiratory effort.

The considerable amount of data generated by PSG is usually summarised graphically (Figure 2.4). Although sophisticated software is often used to analyse sleep stages, the high levels of artefact require a trained technician to manually confirm any computerised analysis.

There are several limitations and controversial issues regarding PSG (Table 2.3).

Protocols to guide which sleep-disordered subjects would merit from full PSG are lacking. Most would recommend PSG in a specialist centre if:

- the condition is likely to be life-long and potentially disabling (e.g. narcolepsy);
- there are atypical features (e.g. sudden onset of possible sleep walking in adulthood with no previous history of similar phenomena in childhood);
- behavioural disturbances during sleep are potentially injurious (e.g. violent REM sleep behaviour disorder);
- attempts to treat a sleep disorder have failed (e.g. persisting daytime sleepiness despite elimination of obstructive apnoeas by CPAP therapy);
- there is likely to be more than one sleep disorder (e.g. periodic limb movements and obstructive sleep apnoea).

An example of a case where PSG recording was helpful in making a diagnosis unsuspected from the history is shown in Box 2.3.

**Table 2.3** Limitations and issues regarding PSG.

| Pitfalls in interpreting PSG | Comments |
| --- | --- |
| Artefacts during recording | There is considerable potential for technical problems to arise during overnight PSG recording; common examples are: electrode placements slipping, movement artefact obscuring other recordings, electrical interference<br>Ideally a technician should be present throughout the recording to monitor and minimise these issues |
| Normal variants | Deciding whether a given parameter is within the normal range can be difficult; the effects of age are considerable and normative data for each age group are not established; deciding whether minor EEG arousals are clinically significant is often debatable; inter-observer differences in scoring PSGs may be significant |
| Inadequate sleep | A subject may sleep particularly poorly in the PSG environment; complex cases are often recorded for two consecutive nights to minimise the disturbing so-called 'first night effect'; paradoxically, some subjects with primary insomnia may sleep particularly well away from the home environment |
| Prior sleep history | The nature and amount of sleep in the days preceding a PSG recording may heavily influence the interpretation of a single overnight recording |
| More than one sleep disorder | Not infrequently, more than one sleep disorder may be revealed (e.g. excessive periodic limb movements and obstructive sleep apnoea); it can be difficult to decide on treatment options and which is the most clinically relevant finding |
| Drug effects | Many drugs may interfere with accurate interpretation of PSG recordings; common examples include the REM sleep suppressant effects of most antidepressants and the potential exaggeration of obstructive sleep apnoeas by sedatives and opiates |

Box 2.3 **Case example in which overnight recording was helpful in establishing a diagnosis of a sleep disorder (periodic limb movements of sleep) that was not suspected from history alone**

A 45-year-old man was referred for assessment of unrefreshing overnight sleep and troublesome daytime sleepiness (Epworth sleep scale score = 14). For several years, despite obtaining at least eight hours sleep every night, he awoke feeling 'groggy'.

There were no clues from his history indicating the cause of his likely poor quality overnight sleep. He was thin and did not snore although lived alone, making the history a little unreliable. He denied restless legs syndrome but was aware his bedclothes were usually disrupted on waking in the morning.

His polysomnogram (Figure B2.3.1) revealed a degree of sleep-onset insomnia and frequent leg movements through the night, most of which were periodic in nature. The movements were associated with pulse rate rises and minor arousals on his EEG.

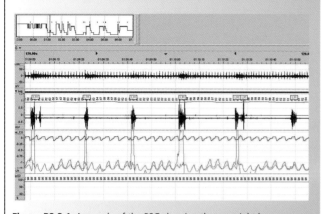

**Figure B2.3.1** A sample of the PSG showing the overnight hypnogram (insert) and a two-minute trace with frequent and regular left leg movements (LM). Breathing parameters were all normal (not shown).

He was diagnosed with periodic limb movement disorder and responded well to a dopamine agonist drug taken before bed.

The PSG was helpful not only in showing his excessive leg movements but also demonstrating they were adversely affecting his sleep continuity and causing minor arousals from sleep.

The majority of parasomnia cases do not require PSG confirmation of the diagnosis if a clear history is obtained. Furthermore, it is rare to obtain useful information from PSG in those with chronic primary insomnia.

## Objective tests of sleepiness and wakefulness

### Sleepiness

There are no truly objective tests that will directly assess a subject's levels of sleepiness. The most widely used surrogate measure is the multiple sleep latency test (MSLT). A subject is asked to lie on a bed fully clothed and encouraged to fall asleep in a sleep-inducing environment whilst monitored. The average latency to fall into stage 1 non-REM sleep is recorded for four or five nap opportunities at two-hourly intervals through the morning and early afternoon. The depth of any sleep obtained is noted and whether or not REM sleep is achieved. Each nap opportunity lasts 20 minutes.

The MSLT is very sensitive to minor procedural variations and a strict protocol is essential. In general, an average sleep latency of 10 minutes or less may be considered abnormal although there is a wide variation in control populations. Perhaps paradoxically, sleep latencies also tend to increase with age even though the elderly are generally viewed as more 'sleepy'. Ideally, the previous night's sleep should be monitored to assess any possible contribution of sleep deprivation. Drugs potentially influencing sleep quality and

quantity should be stopped, if possible, at least a week before the test.

Patients with significant daytime sleepiness will normally have mean sleep latencies of eight minutes or considerably less. In control subjects, one night of sleep deprivation will typically produce a subsequent sleep latency of around three minutes. In narcolepsy, a latency of eight minutes or less with at least two of the naps containing REM sleep within 15 minutes would fulfil the strict diagnostic criteria.

Although considered a 'gold standard', the MSLT should always be interpreted with caution. The wide variation of sleep latencies obtained from MSLTs in the general population often produces both false positive and negative results.

### Wakefulness

In real-life situations, the ability to stay alert is arguably more important to measure or confirm than the ability to fall asleep easily. As with the MSLT, however, deciding an abnormal result can be difficult and normative data for tests assessing wakefulness are lacking.

In drug trials, the maintenance of wakefulness test (MWT) is the most widely used index of wakefulness. As with the MSLT, the subject is asked to recline in a potentially sleep-inducing environment with EEG and video recording. Unlike the MSLT, however, the instruction is to stay awake, usually for 40-minute sessions, subsequently repeated four times. If sleep is witnessed within 15 minutes or so, despite attempts to stay awake, the result may be considered abnormal.

A less labour-intensive test of wakefulness is the Oxford Sleep Resistance (OSLER) test. Usually for four 40-minute sessions, a subject has to respond manually on a button to a regularly flashing light. Lack of any motor response for seven consecutive three-second intervals is recorded as a sleep episode. Shorter periods of

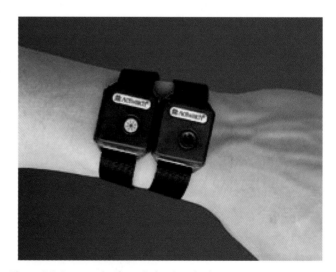

**Figure 2.5** An example of a typical actigraph. The person is wearing two varieties of a commonly used device.

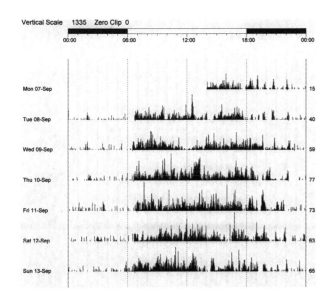

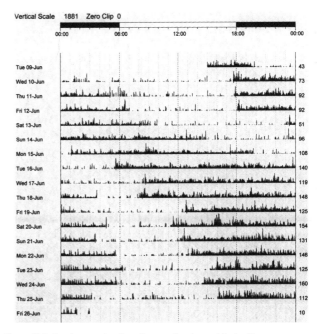

**Figure 2.6** An example of a normal actigraph recording taken over one week. Time of day is shown at the top of the graph. The lines indicate the levels of arm movement and imply a regular waking time of 06:30 with lessening activity levels during the evening. Overnight, movement is minimal, between 23:00 and 06:30.

unresponsiveness indicate impaired vigilance possibly secondary to 'microsleeps'. There appear to be good correlations between sleep latencies obtained by the OSLER test and the MWT.

## Actigraphy

Actigraphs are small devices resembling a wristwatch that record small movements, usually at the wrist, when a subject is presumed to be awake (Figure 2.5). Recordings can be made over a period of weeks and a profile obtained of the sleep'wake cycle (Figure 2.6).

A large amount of data is gathered and modern devices will also record parameters such as audio signals, light levels and pulse rate.

Using movement as a surrogate measure for wakefulness is clearly prone to providing false positive and negative data but actigraphy is an inexpensive and unobtrusive technique. It is most useful in confirming diary information on sleep–wake cycles and also in investigating possible disorders of circadian timing (Figure 2.7).

**Figure 2.7** An abnormal actigraph recording in a subject with a rare abnormality of circadian timing. It demonstrates a tendency to sleep an hour later each day through the two weeks of recording. This helps to diagnose non-24-hour sleep phase syndrome in which a subject has an internal clock that runs on approximately 25 hours a day rather than 24 hours. This is most commonly seen in individuals who are blind from birth and unable to entrain their clock mechanisms to the day–night cycle via pathways from the retina to the hypothalamus.

## Further reading

American Academy of Sleep Medicine (2005) *International classification of sleep disorders: diagnostic and coding manual*, 2nd edition. American Academy of Sleep Medicine, Westchester, IL.

Ancoli-Israel, S., Cole, R., Alessi, C. *et al.* (2003) The role of actigraphy in the study of sleep and circadian rhythms. *Sleep*, **26**, 343–392.

Carskadon, M.A., Dement, W.C., Mitler, M.M. *et al.* (1986) Guidelines for the Multiple Sleep Latency Test (MSLT): A standard measure of sleepiness. *Sleep*, **9**, 519–524.

Keenan, S.A. (1992) Polysomnography: technical aspects in adolescents and adults. *J Clin Neurophysiol*, **9**, 21–31.

Raymond, B., Cayton, R.M. and Chappell, M.J. (2003) Combined index of heart rate variability and oximetry in screening for the sleep apnoea/ hypopnoea syndrome. *J Sleep Res*, **12**, 53–61.

# CHAPTER 3

# Excessive Daytime Sleepiness

## Introduction

Around 5% of the adult population experiences a level of daytime sleepiness that could be considered abnormal and potentially intrusive or even dangerous to routine daily activities. Complaints of drowsiness or an inappropriate and excessive tendency to nap during the day need to be carefully distinguished from simple 'tiredness', 'fatigue' or 'lack of energy'. These phenomena usually

*ABC of Sleep Medicine*, First Edition. Paul Reading.
© 2013 John Wiley & Sons, Ltd. Published 2013 by John Wiley & Sons, Ltd.

have different aetiologies, such as chronic fatigue syndrome in which there is no objective evidence for an increased tendency to fall asleep.

When severe, excessive daytime sleepiness (EDS) should be treated as a potentially serious disability affecting most activities of daily living. Indeed, young subjects with EDS usually struggle to achieve their full potential, especially if untreated.

Unfortunately, EDS can still be dismissed by many as resulting merely from poor lifestyle habits, laziness or reduced motivation. In the past, EDS has even been considered as a 'moral failing'. Consequently, the associated symptoms of poor concentration, motor clumsiness and automatic behaviours are frequently not recognised or, at best, misdiagnosed. Furthermore, EDS is often mistakenly attributed to reflect mood disorder (depression), hormonal balance (hypothyroidism) or anaemia, even though none of these typically produces EDS directly.

Formal diagnosis of a sleep disorder causing EDS may be delayed in youngsters who display behavioural problems of irritability or paradoxical hyperactivity rather than more obvious symptoms of sleepiness. Furthermore, teenagers and young adults, in particular, may seek to 'self-medicate' with recreational stimulant drugs. Potentially, this may also confuse or delay any underlying medical diagnosis and treatment.

The potential hazards of EDS when performing monotonous tasks such as driving are obvious and often preventable. Occupational health physicians are increasingly aware of EDS as an issue both at work and on the daily commute, especially in shift workers.

When caused by a sleep disorder, EDS is usually a persistent or chronic symptom although there are a few rare causes of intermittent sleepiness.

The term 'hypersomnolence' is virtually synonymous with EDS although strictly it refers to abnormally increased sleep time over the full 24-hour period. Importantly, some causes of EDS simply reflect sleepiness at unconventional times either because the sleep–wake cycle is dysregulated (e.g. narcolepsy) or because of abnormal circadian timing (e.g. jet lag). In these situations, total sleep time over the day–night cycle is usually of normal duration.

The physical signs of EDS are often subtle and may go unrecognised, particularly in the elderly, making a good history from the subject and close contacts particularly important. Slow eye blinking, yawning and brief spells of inattention ('microsleeps'), even with eyes open, may be observable manifestations of EDS. Slurred speech, impaired fine motor control, resembling drunkenness and even personality change are apparent in severe cases.

## Causes

The commonest cause of mild sleepiness is simply insufficient nocturnal sleep. Variably, this can reflect lifestyle choices, commitments through work or a poor quality sleeping environment. It can be surprising, however, how some subjects complaining of EDS do not appreciate the vital need for most to have around seven hours sleep at night, regarding it as a dispensable commodity. Such subjects typically report worsening EDS as the working week progresses and their 'sleep debt' mounts. Relative improvement in symptoms at weekends or on holiday with extended sleep periods would also be expected. It can occasionally be useful to obtain sleep diaries over a few weeks to demonstrate this pattern.

Aside from insufficient sleep, the causes of EDS can be broadly divided into three categories (Figure 3.1):

1  The commonest reason for significant EDS is poor quality sleep due to a chronic condition such as obstructive sleep apnoea. Subjects may experience a normal or even excessive amount of overnight sleep but are not restored or refreshed in the morning in a manner resembling simple sleep deprivation. Importantly, many drugs may also worsen the quality of sleep even though they produce drowsiness and may extend actual sleep time.

2  Primary sleep disorders in which there is proven or assumed central nervous system pathology accounting for EDS are extremely important to recognise, even though they only account for around 2% of 'sleepy' cases presenting to physicians. Such cases tend not to improve with the passage of time.

3  The third category refers to abnormal timing of a subject's circadian rhythm due to extrinsic or intrinsic 'clock' factors.

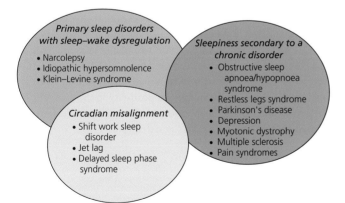

**Figure 3.1** The causes of excessive daytime sleepiness (EDS) in patients seeking medical help may be divided into three main categories. Chronic disorders interfering with sleep quality form the biggest group by far. However, approximately 1 in 50 of subjects with EDS may have a primary sleep disorder such as narcolepsy. Circadian misalignment is an increasingly recognised cause of EDS. The categories are not mutually exclusive and may interact.

In practice, insufficient sleep due to work or social factors (e.g. noisy environment) is the commonest cause of mild EDS.

## Narcolepsy

Narcolepsy has been recognised as a distinct syndrome for well over a century although it is only in the last decade that its underlying neurobiology has been established. Genetic analysis of a canine model of narcolepsy led to the surprising discovery that classical cases of human narcolepsy arise from specific destruction of a few thousand neurons in the lateral hypothalamus. This produces a deficiency of a neuropeptide called hypocretin (alternatively, orexin), a key regulator of the sleep–wake cycle. Although unproven, a variety of evidence suggests that the subtle neurological damage in narcolepsy has an autoimmune basis, occasionally with a defined precipitant such as a viral infection or vaccination.

Narcolepsy most frequently starts in early adolescence and is a life-long affliction. Given its specific neurochemical basis, it is perhaps not surprising that there is a spectrum of severity such that mild cases often escape medical attention. It probably affects as many as 1 in 3000 of Caucasian populations.

The most usual symptom of concern in narcolepsy is an inability to sustain useful alertness for more than about three hours. Irresistible sleep episodes, occasionally without recognising the prior imperative to sleep, may produce 'sleep attacks' in inappropriate situations and at any time of day. Naps are typically fairly short (around 20 minutes or less) and often refreshing. Many narcoleptics can sustain wakefulness if engaged in alerting activities but fight sleep if bored or unoccupied. Few can watch films without napping. Aside from frank sleep episodes, most will describe frequent so-called 'microsleeps' in which full awareness is diminished and automatic behaviours may occur with poor recall.

It is often not appreciated how badly narcoleptics sleep at night. Normal sleep architecture is generally disorganised, particularly during REM sleep periods which are fragmented and often intermixed with partial wakefulness. This produces vivid and often disturbing dreams at sleep–wake transitions, potentially confused with reality. Elements of REM sleep such as paralysis of voluntary muscles can also intrude into wakefulness, even at sleep onset. This symptom of sleep paralysis is not specific, however, and is commonly reported as an occasional disturbing phenomenon in normal populations.

The fragmented sleep of many narcoleptics almost certainly contributes to EDS and may merit specific drug therapy. Furthermore, virtually every parasomnia, including sleep walking and dream enactment (REM sleep behaviour disorder), can be seen more commonly in narcoleptics. In addition, other sleep disorders, notably obstructive sleep apnoea, may co-exist with narcolepsy and should not be overlooked, especially if symptom control appears to deteriorate with time.

By far the most specific and diagnostically important symptom in narcolepsy is cataplexy. This unusual phenomenon reflects the intrusion of REM sleep paralysis during wakefulness, most often when the subject is experiencing or expecting a positive emotion such as laughter or pleasant surprise. Attacks are generally brief and take a few seconds to build up, typically with head bobbing or facial jerking at the onset. This may suggest an epileptic phenomenon although a key feature of cataplexy is maintained awareness of the environment even when paralysed. Partial attacks are common and may be confined to slurred speech, transient neck flexion or sagging of the knees.

Rarely, cataplexy is the most troublesome symptom with numerous attacks each day, triggered by a range of emotions or situations. However, it is relatively rare for medical practitioners to witness cataplexy, as it usually occurs in relaxed circumstances with family or friends. It should be noted that over 30% of narcoleptics either have no symptoms of cataplexy or only very occasional episodes.

## Investigations

Narcolepsy remains largely a clinical diagnosis based on a full history (Table 3.1). However, investigations may help to confirm clinical impressions and exclude other diagnoses. International guidelines have rightly placed great emphasis on the presence of typical cataplexy which, if present, in the context of EDS is sufficient for a positive diagnosis. Many authorities, however, would advocate obtaining objective evidence of sleepiness by undertaking

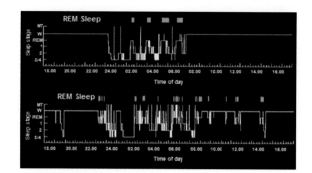

**Figure 3.2** 24-hour hypnograms showing the distribution of wake and sleep across a full day and night for a control subject (top) and a narcoleptic (bottom). In the narcoleptic, there is a chaotic distribution of sleep across the night with frequent arousals. During the day there are several brief sleep episodes with REM sleep intrusions.

a multiple sleep latency test (MSLT). Over four or five nap opportunities at two-hourly intervals, a narcoleptic should fall asleep, on average, within eight minutes or sooner and enter REM sleep within 15 minutes in at least two of the naps. These criteria have some validity although are very dependent on how the investigation is undertaken, its rigour and the precise protocol used. For example, monitoring of overnight sleep to ensure adequate sleep length before the MSLT is mandatory but often overlooked.

Overnight polysomnography in narcolepsy usually reveals poorly organised and fragmented sleep, often with an excess of movement, both in REM and non-REM sleep stages (Figure 3.2). An early onset of REM sleep within 20 minutes might also be seen. These changes are not specific, however, and may be influenced by concomitant medication.

The levels of the deficient neuropeptide hypocretin (orexin) can be measured in cerebrospinal fluid (CSF) samples from a lumbar puncture although this remains a highly specialised investigation. Disappointingly, in cases where there is doubt about the diagnosis, the test is rarely useful given that hypocretin deficiency is usually only seen clearly in clinically obvious cases with typical cataplexy.

The remarkably tight association of the human leucocyte antigen (HLA) DQB1*0602 with typical narcolepsy (around 95% are positive for this antigen) has been used to justify HLA typing. However, most authorities rarely recommend this approach given the relatively high prevalence of antigen positivity in the general population (around 25%). Furthermore, the association is less marked for atypical or rare familial cases of narcolepsy.

## Treatment

Most narcoleptics benefit from drug medication although planned brief naps during the day or adjustments to diet can improve symptom control in many. Caffeinated drinks or caffeine supplements from pharmacies are rarely sufficient to provide normal alertness but can be a useful supplement. It should be emphasised that, even with optimal drug treatment, a significant proportion of patients are never normalised with respect to their sleep–wake cycle.

The commoner options for drug treatment are shown in Table 3.2. EDS is usually the most disabling symptom and combinations of wake-promoting agents, typically modafinil and

**Table 3.1** A summary of questions that might help in diagnosing narcolepsy clinically.

| Probe for possible narcolepsy | Comments |
| --- | --- |
| Have you fallen asleep in particularly unusual situations? | Most narcoleptics will admit to unplanned naps in public, on buses for example. |
| Are you prone to losing objects around the house or performing inappropriate behaviours when 'half asleep'? | Automatic behaviours during presumed 'microsleeps' are very common alongside frank sleep episodes |
| Do you find short naps restoring? | In contrast to many causes of severe EDS, narcoleptics often find a 20-minute nap restorative, allowing them a further period of useful wakefulness |
| Do you routinely dream in short daytime naps? | A positive answer implies that REM sleep is occurring soon after sleep onset, a very characteristic feature of narcolepsy |
| In general, are your dreams very vivid, bizarre or difficult to distinguish from reality? | Most narcoleptics report unusual or excessive dream activity with an unusually clear and persisting memory for vivid dreams or nightmares |
| Is your overnight sleep fragmented and of poor quality? | The majority of narcolepsy patients sleep very poorly overnight, either with spontaneous awakenings or intrusions of REM sleep phenomena and other parasomnias |
| Do you experience brief symptoms of weakness when emotional, particularly during laughter? | A very important question for exploring cataplexy which can be focal or subtle and confined to speech disturbance or head bobbing |
| Have you developed a craving for sweet foods in particular, perhaps overnight? | Increasingly, it is recognised that narcolepsy is associated with unusual eating habits or appetite control |

**Table 3.2** A summary of drug therapy typically used in narcolepsy.

| Symptom | Drug | Dose | Comments |
|---|---|---|---|
| Excessive sleepiness | Modafinil | 100–400 mg daily; usually in two doses | Typically taken after waking and around noon. Side effects usually mild (headache and gastric upset) |
| | | | Slight increase in blood pressure possible, needs monitoring |
| | | | Enzyme induction, so care needed with contraceptive pill |
| | Dexamphetamine | 10–60 mg daily; taken through the day in 5 or 10 mg doses | Generally a second-line treatment to modafinil but often used as an 'add on' Monitor for side effects such as hypertension and agitation |
| | | | Abuse potential appears low in narcoleptic population |
| | Methylphenidate | 20–60 mg daily; taken through the day in 10 or 20 mg doses | Similar pharmacological profile to amphetamine although slightly longer lasting |
| | Selegiline | 10–40 mg daily; usually in two doses | Metabolised to amphetamine Can be used (off licence) as a mild stimulant in doses higher than those for Parkinson's disease |
| Cataplexy | Venlafaxine | 75–225 mg daily: usually one dose long-acting preparations | An antidepressant that supresses REM sleep, raising the threshold for cataplexy |
| | Clomipramine | 20–75 mg daily; usually in one or two doses | Often effective but side effects of weight gain and dry mouth may limit use |
| | Sodium oxybate | 4.5–9 g nightly; taken before bed and typically at 02:00 a.m., if awake | Good trial data suggest cataplexy may reduce by 90%; Other symptoms of narcolepsy, including sleepiness, may also improve; Short half-life leads to few 'hangover' effects; Expense and fear over misuse limit practical use |
| Disrupted overnight sleep | Clonazepam or alternative hypnotic | Standard doses | Justified as a long-term treatment if sleep disruption a prominent symptom. Even if sleep maintenance improved, sleep quality not always enhanced |
| | | | Care needed if co-morbid sleep apnoea a possibility |
| | Sodium oxybate | 4.5–9 g nightly | Usually improves sleep quality and daytime sleepiness. Avoid with alcohol as respiratory depression a risk |

dexamphetamine, may be needed. Cataplexy may improve concurrently with increased wakefulness but approximately 50% of patients benefit from additional medication. The commonest strategy relies on using antidepressant drugs, the majority of which suppress the tendency to enter REM sleep by increasing brain levels of catecholamines such as serotonin and noradrenaline.

If nocturnal sleep is particularly disturbed, non-specific hypnotic agents such as clonazepam may usefully improve sleep continuity although rarely improve its overall quality. Significant sleep paralysis, hallucinations or other REM sleep-related nocturnal phenomena may also improve with antidepressant treatment as in cataplexy.

The best controlled evidence for treating narcolepsy is available for sodium oxybate, a liquid preparation usually given in divided doses before bed and once through the night. It is short-acting and strongly promotes deep non-REM sleep as its main action. It improves all the core symptoms of narcolepsy although the mechanism of action in cataplexy remains obscure. It is a controversial drug, largely due to its commercial expense and fears over potential misuse recreationally.

## Secondary narcolepsy

With increasing knowledge of sleep neurobiology and the nature of narcolepsy, it is valid to consider secondary causes, especially if there is proven pathology in the region of the hypothalamus. Brain imaging may therefore be justified in certain situations, particularly if narcoleptic symptoms are atypical. Very occasionally, inflammatory disorders such as multiple sclerosis may be associated with a form of narcolepsy with lesions seen in or around the hypothalamus on imaging. A variety of structural pathologies in the region of the floor of the third ventricle, adjacent to the hypothalamus, have also been reported to cause narcoleptic symptoms (Figure 3.3).

In a range of neurological disorders, the level and nature of EDS may mimic narcolepsy even if the underlying mechanism remains obscure. Examples include myotonic dystrophy, Parkinson's disease, head injury and certain rare developmental disorders, such as Prader–Willi syndrome. In selected cases, wake-promoting therapy may be justified, assuming more common causes of EDS have been addressed.

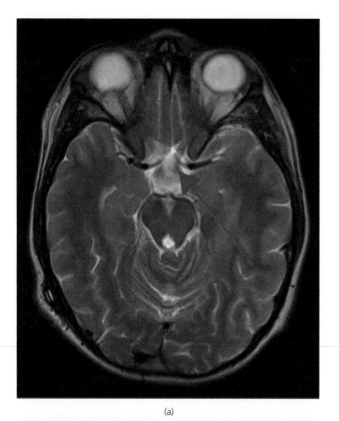

(a)

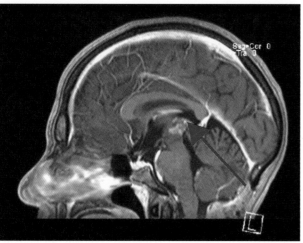

(b)

**Figure 3.3** MR brain scans, (a) axial and (b) sagittal views, of a 20-year-old man who developed severe sleepiness resembling a form of narcolepsy after removal of a low grade tumour (glioma) in the region of the third ventricle. The arrows show abnormal signal indicating post-operative scar tissue (gliosis) predominantly in the posterior hypothalamus.

## Idiopathic hypersomnolence

A rare cause of severe EDS often affecting young populations and potentially mimicking narcolepsy is idiopathic hypersomnolence (IH). The underlying neurobiology is not established and subjects simply appear to need far more sleep than average. In typical cases, despite 10 hours of good quality sleep, there are major difficulties

**Table 3.3** Some clinical features typical for idiopathic hypersomnolence (IH).

| Symptoms typical in IH | Comment |
| --- | --- |
| Unavoidable daytime naps | Naps tend to be long and unrefreshing but otherwise unremarkable (e.g. no dream phenomena) |
| Automatic behaviours common | There is usually reduced alertness throughout the day such that some behaviours are performed on 'autopilot' and not recalled |
| Overnight sleep is prolonged | Sleep quality and quantity appear normal or even better than average when formally measured by investigations |
| Morning waking difficult | Often the most disabling symptom with subjects appearing 'confused' or irritable if awoken at a conventional hour |
| Mood disorder common | If present, this probably is more likely a consequence rather a cause of the excessive sleepiness |
| Sleep latency is around eight minutes or less on a multiple sleep latency test (MSLT) | In a 20-minute nap opportunity, subjects with IH usually fall into deep non-REM sleep but not REM sleep |

arising at a conventional hour and a subsequent propensity for prolonged unrefreshing daytime naps. Unlike narcolepsy, there are few symptoms suggesting abnormal REM sleep or related phenomena (Table 3.3).

In some patients the clinical picture appears to lie between IH and narcolepsy. Given that treatment options with daytime stimulants are broadly similar in both conditions, the distinction may be considered somewhat academic. However, in general, wake-promoting treatments tend to be less successful in IH, with many patients unable to work or study effectively. Frustration and depression are frequent associations.

## Circadian misalignment

Jet lag is an obvious example of how the normal circadian influences on sleep propensity are poorly synchronised with the light–dark cycle after travelling across time zones. The EDS and insomnia associated with jet lag are usually associated with minor gastroenterological symptoms reflecting how the functions of other organs also have internal rhythmicity. Travel eastwards produces more symptoms, since most people find it more difficult to advance their internal clocks to local time.

Shift work, particularly involving a rotating schedule, is a common and overlooked source of significant hypersomnolence. Although many younger people appear to adapt well, the ability to obtain quality recovery sleep during the day after night shifts diminishes with increasing age. The consequent chronic sleep deprivation associated with shift work has been associated with a variety of health problems, including increased cancer risk, particularly in females.

With genetic advances and increasing scientific knowledge of the subcellular internal clock mechanism, a number of intrinsic circadian dysrhythmias are now recognised. The commonest is delayed sleep phase syndrome in which a subject is unable to sleep before 1:00 a.m. or later. Once asleep, sleep quality appears sound and is of normal length if permitted. Arising at a conventional early hour for work or education is invariably the main adverse consequence. This tends to affect teenagers and is often inappropriately dismissed simply as a lifestyle issue.

Rarer 'clock problems' are advanced sleep phase syndrome and non-24 hour sleep phase syndrome. A specific mutation of a clock gene has been discovered to explain the former, in which subjects arise from sleep abnormally early having been unable to stay awake beyond 8:00 p.m. The latter problem is most often seen in congenitally blind subjects who are unable to adjust their circadian rhythms precisely to 24 hours using external light cues.

Treating circadian misalignment is often pragmatic, particularly when due to extrinsic factors. However, if there is a desire to control or advance the time of sleep onset, a low dose of melatonin (0.5 mg) taken two hours before bed may help.

## Further reading

Akerstedt, T. (1998) Shift work and disturbed sleep/wakefulness. *Sleep Med Rev*, **2**, 117–128.

Bassetti, C. and Aldrich, M.S. (1997) Idiopathic hypersomnia. A series of 42 patients. *Brain*, **120**, 1423–1435.

Billiard, M., Bassetti, C., Dauvilliers, Y. *et al.* (2006) EFNS guidelines on management of narcolepsy. *Eur J Neurol*, **13**, 1035–1048.

Dauvilliers, Y., Arnulf, I. and Mignot, E. (2007) Narcolepsy with cataplexy. *Lancet*, **369**, 499–511.

Sack, R.L. and Lewy, A.J. (2001) Circadian rhythm disorders: lessons from the blind. *Sleep Med Rev*, **5**, 189–206.

# CHAPTER 4

# Sleep Apnoea Syndromes

## OVERVIEW

- Obstructive sleep apnoea (OSA) syndrome most commonly develops on the background of severe snoring and affects around 4% of middle-aged males
- Most, but not all, patients with OSA have significant central obesity affecting abdominal and neck girth
- The most obvious consequence of OSA syndrome is unrefreshing overnight sleep with significant subsequent daytime somnolence, predisposing to accidents and poor work performance
- Increasingly, the adverse metabolic and cardiovascular effects of OSA on general health are recognised as potentially reversible phenomena
- Continuous positive airways pressure (CPAP) therapy is the best proven treatment for OSA although alternative approaches are available if it is unsuccessful or inappropriate
- Mandibular advancement devices may be successful in mild or moderate OSA
- Central sleep apnoea (CSA) occurs when subjects fail to initiate breathing when asleep and has a variety of causes and associations, most notably significant heart failure
- Treatment of CSA is complex and may not always be necessary if there are no adverse daytime consequences

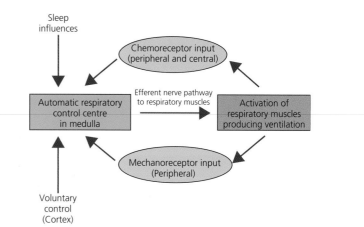

**Figure 4.1** Factors involved in the respiratory control system.

It is perhaps unfortunate that snoring is often perceived as something of a laughing or trivial matter. However, very severe snorers may obstruct their airways so frequently as to partially arouse them from sleep over 500 times a night, thereby ruining sleep quality and potentially causing life-threatening daytime drowsiness. The secondary adverse effects of sleep-disordered breathing on daytime performance, cognition, quality of life, mood and general medical health, as well as the sleep efficiency of bed partners, are increasingly recognised.

At least a third of middle-aged males snore habitually, with around 10% producing noise levels potentially audible in adjacent rooms. Although prevalence figures vary across populations, up to 3% of males and 2% of females over 50 may have obstructive sleep apnoea syndrome (OSAS), an important and eminently treatable condition.

During sleep, the control of breathing is involuntary, regulated by an automatic negative feedback system, largely centred in the lower brainstem (Figure 4.1). The medullary control centre receives information about acidity and gas concentrations from chemoreceptors situated both in the brain itself and in carotid arteries. A number of mechanoreceptors from the respiratory tract and muscle spindles in respiratory muscles also influence the system.

In general, breathing in sleep is shallower and the normal homeostatic set points, such as carbon dioxide levels, are less tightly controlled. This occurs particularly during the REM sleep stage, in which respiratory rates become variable.

In normal breathing, air is sucked into the lungs by creating a negative pressure in the upper airways during inspiration. The tendency for the airway to close off is counteracted by persistent or tonic stiffness in muscles, such as the genioglossus and surrounding palate. As sleep deepens, these areas naturally become floppier causing the airway to narrow, potentially producing air turbulence (heard as snoring) or frank obstruction of breathing. A useful analogy refers to the difficulty encountered when drinking through an old-fashioned paper straw. If the straw becomes wet, it collapses on itself, initially causing 'slurping' before complete obstruction. Further attempts to suck harder are counterproductive.

*ABC of Sleep Medicine*, First Edition. Paul Reading.
© 2013 John Wiley & Sons, Ltd. Published 2013 by John Wiley & Sons, Ltd.

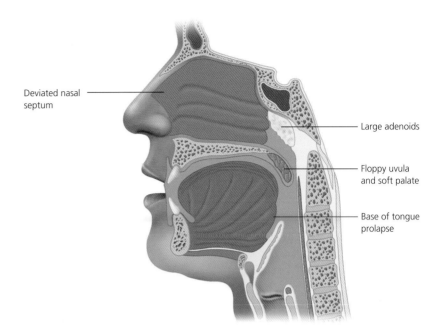

Deviated nasal septum

Large adenoids

Floppy uvula and soft palate

Base of tongue prolapse

**Figure 4.2** Possible sites causing snoring.

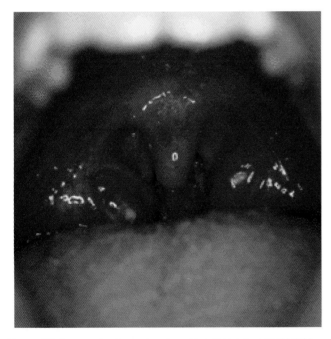

**Figure 4.3** An example of severely enlarged tonsils in a six-year-old child with sleep apnoea.

Anatomically determining precisely where the airway obstructs in a snoring subject can be difficult unless there are clear visible physical factors, such as enlarged nasal polyps, adenoids or tonsils (Figures 4.2). The latter are particularly common in children between two and six years of age (Figure 4.3).

An apnoea is arbitrarily defined as cessation of breathing for at least 10 seconds and will quickly lead to hypoxia and a rise in plasma carbon dioxide levels (hypercapnia). If due to obstruction, the detection of these physiological changes automatically leads to increased respiratory effort, sympathetic activation and partial arousal from sleep which may not be registered or recalled consciously by the subject.

In a small proportion of subjects with sleep apnoea, the problem arises because there is reduced or an absent effort to breathe, so-called central sleep apnoea (CSA).

Hypopneas occur when there is partial occlusion enough to reduce airflow by 30% and oxyhaemoglobin levels by 4%, again over a 10-second interval. The apnoea-hypopnea index (AHI) refers to the number of events per hour and is a commonly used measure describing the severity of sleep-disordered breathing. An AHI of 10–20 roughly corresponds to mild sleep apnoea whereas a figure over 50 generally produces severe symptoms. However, OSAS remains a clinical diagnosis and an apparently high AHI may not be clinically significant unless there are adverse daytime consequences, particularly on wakefulness and performance.

## Diagnosing obstructive sleep apnoea

Obstructive sleep apnoea causes a variety of symptoms and can, therefore, present to clinicians in a number of ways (Table 4.1). Given its high and increasing prevalence, there should always be a low threshold for considering it. A number of nocturnal neurological problems, including cluster headaches and epilepsy, are associated with OSA and will often improve with successful treatment of the breathing disorder.

OSA predominantly affects males who have central obesity (Figure 4.4), typically with collar sizes above 17 inches. However, many other factors may predispose an individual to OSA (Table 4.2). In females, for unclear reasons, equivalent levels of OSA may carry a worse prognosis compared to male subjects.

OSA may also be overlooked in those who sleep alone and a snoring history is absent. OSA should therefore always be considered in anyone who feels significantly unrefreshed after an apparently adequate period of nocturnal sleep.

**Table 4.1** Various symptoms commonly associated with obstructive sleep apnoea.

| Waking symptoms | Nocturnal symptoms |
|---|---|
| Excessive sleepiness or fatigue | Snoring |
| Morning headache or 'fullness' | Choking or witnessed apnoeas |
| Poor concentration and attention | Restless sleep |
| Cognitive dysfunction | Sleep maintenance insomnia |
| Personality change | Nocturia |
| Poor work performance | Sweating |
| Erectile dysfunction, reduced libido | Dry mouth through night |
| Sore throat | Acid reflux |

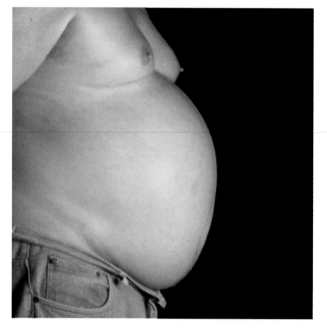

**Figure 4.4** A typical physical phenotype of a male subject with OSA.

**Table 4.2** Factors predisposing to obstructive sleep apnoea.

| Factor | Cause | Comment |
|---|---|---|
| Small upper airway | Obesity | Particularly central obesity in those who are 'apple-shaped'; increased neck collar size is clearest risk factor |
| | Tobacco smoking | Possibly inflamed upper airways |
| | Hormonal factors | Hypothyroidism and acromegaly may increase soft tissue around airway; post-menopausal women more at risk |
| | Supine position | Snoring generally worse when sleeping on back; a pillow wedged between the shoulders may prevent sleeping in a supine position |
| | Upper airway lesions | Rhinitis, nasal polyps, enlarged tonsils/adenoids may produce OSA in non-obese subjects |
| | Retrognathia or facial deformity | A severely receding chin, either as a normal variant or as part of a developmental syndrome, may increase risk |
| Reduced dilator activity of upper airways muscles | Sedative drugs or anaesthetics | Alcohol and benzodiazepines are common examples |
| | Neurological disorders | Any cause of bulbar muscle weakness; significant strokes commonly produce OSA in early stages of recovery |
| Increased chest wall resistance | Obesity | Severe truncal obesity or increased muscle mass in bodybuilders may simply 'weigh down' the chest during sleep |

Aside from unrefreshing overnight sleep and daytime somnolence, OSA has been linked as an independent contributor to a variety of metabolic and cardiovascular long-term problems (Table 4.3). Many of these presumably occur because the sympathetic arousal systems are persistently activated overnight, although a number may simply reflect the adverse consequences of chronic severe sleep deprivation. The latter may even lead to an impression of significant cognitive decline or even dementia.

The commonest method for diagnosing OSA is through simple home oximetry using a finger probe to detect plasma oxygen desaturations and pulse rate through the night (Chapter 2). A typical positive recording is shown with pulse rate rises accompanying the dips in oxygen levels (Figure 2.3). This is a relatively inexpensive procedure and is useful for monitoring treatment effects.

With oximetry, false positive results may be obtained if oxygen dips are secondary to central sleep apnoea (CSA) and not simple obstruction of the airway. Furthermore, chronic respiratory disease producing chronic hypoxaemia may complicate interpretation. The procedure is also prone to artefacts and will not demonstrate

the poor sleep quality of those heavy snorers who do not fully obstruct their breathing but are partially awoken by the increased breathing effort. Such a concept of an 'upper airways resistance syndrome' (UARS) is controversial but almost certainly is valid for some subjects.

Depending on resources, suspected cases of OSA in whom oximetry has not been helpful or fully diagnostic may proceed to further overnight investigations. Ambulatory devices are increasingly available and allow recordings at home of several useful parameters. These include oxygen saturations, pulse rate, nasal airflow, respiratory effort deduced from pressure transducers on chest and abdominal surfaces, and leg movements. The last measure may indicate excessive and regular limb restlessness as an additional cause for poor sleep quality.

Full polysomography in a sleep laboratory is sometimes justified to quantify and stage overnight sleep accurately in order to assess the presence and potential contribution of additional sleep disorders.

**Table 4.3** Proposed clinical adverse consequences of OSA.

| Possible adverse consequence | Comment |
| --- | --- |
| Hypertension | A link with hypertension has been clearly established, particularly overnight when blood pressure normally falls significantly |
| Increased diabetic risk | Increased insulin resistance in OSA has been proven although the precise mechanism remains obscure |
| Obesity | Increased resistance to chemical satiety signals in the brain (notably leptin) has been proposed |
| Hormonal changes | Associated endocrine abnormalities often seen although causation not always established; reduced growth hormone secretion in children with severe OSA is probably a significant clinical consequences |
| Impaired inflammatory response | The sleep deprivation associated with chronic OSA may lead to less effective vaccinations and increased susceptibility to infections |
| Increased cancer risk | A theoretical risk, possibly related to chronic sleep deprivation and reduced immune surveillance |
| Increased brain atrophy | Several large studies have shown reduced grey matter throughout most of the cortex and in part of the cerebellum of severe OSA patients; the mechanism is not established |

**Table 4.4** Reasons for discontinuing CPAP therapy.

| Complication of CPAP therapy potentially leading to discontinuation | Corrective measure |
| --- | --- |
| Air leak | Change mask or headgear; try chin strap; consider full face mask |
| Nasal symptoms | Heated water humidification; minimise mouth leak; consider inhaled steroids |
| Skin ulceration | Change mask type; protect skin |
| Claustrophobia | Use smaller mask or nasal seals |
| Aerophagy | Reduce pressure or usage of CPAP |
| Noise of CPAP | Reassure; ear plugs |
| Lack of efficacy on daytime symptoms | Check pressures and repeat oximetry; diagnosis may be incorrect |

## Treating obstructive sleep apnoea

The aims of treating OSA are to improve overnight sleep quality and daytime sleepiness, reduce the risk of accidents and minimise the associated medical complications such as hypertension.

### Initial approaches in general practice

- Obese patients should be encouraged strongly to lose weight, especially if recent weight gain has coincided with an increase in shirt collar size. Arguably, there should be a lower threshold for recommending anti-obesity drugs or bariatric surgery to aid weight loss in the presence of significant OSA. A 10% loss in weight might be expected to reduce the AHI by 25% in an average subject.
- Advice should also be given regarding smoking cessation and excessive alcohol intake.
- Sedating drugs, especially benzodiazepines, should be withdrawn if possible.
- Nasal dilators may improve snoring but rarely improve frank OSA. Inhaled steroids are recommended if there is evidence for rhinitis or nasal polyps.
- It is difficult to alter sleeping posture but physical attempts to avoid rolling over into a supine position are sometimes successful.

## Nasal continuous positive airway pressure (CPAP)

In those with established OSAS on the basis of overnight investigations and daytime symptoms, nasal CPAP is now regarded as first-line treatment assuming conservative measures have failed. Nasal CPAP delivers air at increased pressure through inspiration and expiration, acting as a pneumatic splint, gently forcing the airway more open.

A variety of pumps and nasal or full face silicon masks are now available to suit different head shapes and individual preferences. The simplest system uses a fixed pressure of air (typically 6–20 cm $H_2O$) delivered through the night. Some systems are programmed to increase the pressure over the first 30 minutes of sleep if sleep onset is rendered difficult. Other machines have a variable pressure setting and can be used to auto-titrate the correct pressure, aiming to eliminate over 90% of obstructive episodes. A variable pressure or auto-set system is usually better tolerated but more expensive.

The majority of CPAP machines have an internal clock to measure average usage overnight. Unfortunately, long-term compliance is rarely above 50%. Reasons for discontinuation are variable (Table 4.4) and are inversely proportional to the level of education and support available to the patients. In general, the more severe the level of OSA, the more likely the subject is to obtain symptom relief and, therefore, persist with therapy.

## Mechanical devices to keep airway open
### Mandibular advancement or positioning devices (MADs)

These hold the mandible and hyoid forwards and can be effective in mild or moderate OSA, especially if the obstruction is mainly at the base of the tongue. They advance the mandible to about 75% of its maximum protruding position, at least 50 mm forward. The devices are constructed either of one piece, similar to a gum shield, or of two pieces that are adjustable and usually require fitting by a dental surgeon. The latter are harder, less bulky and generally better tolerated.

MADs cannot be used in subjects who are edentulous or who have had extensive dental procedures. They are less effective in severe obesity or in those with temporo-mandibular joint dysfunction.

### Other devices

Nasal dilators can be internal or external and may help with snoring. They rarely improve established OSA, however.

Palatal inserts to stiffen the uvula and palate have been developed. Evidence for efficacy has yet to be established.

Devices to keep the tongue anchored by suction to the anterior part of the mouth tend not to be tolerated. Excessive salivation and soreness usually limit usefulness.

### Palatal and tongue surgery

Although a single surgical procedure to widen the airway may seem a relatively simple and attractive approach, it has become increasingly unpopular as a treatment option. With the exception of adeno-tonsillectomy, usually in children, long-term results of surgery are extremely variable, partly because it is often difficult to accurately determine the site of obstruction. Furthermore, the notion that resulting scar tissue will stiffen the palate and help reduce compliance has not been substantiated.

Either uvulo-palatoplasty or tongue resection can be achieved by both conventional surgery and laser or radiofrequency techniques. However, these procedures are rarely successful in severe OSA and are associated with considerable post-operative morbidity. If CPAP therapy is used subsequent to such surgery, mouth leaks are common and necessitate wearing a full face mask.

Particularly in children with lower jaw or facial deformity, orthognathic surgery to expand the maxilla and advance the mandible may be appropriate. This approach is highly specialised and requires detailed pre-operative assessment with imaging.

### Wake-promoting drugs

Approximately 5% of subjects with significant OSA fail to respond to best available or first-line treatments such as CPAP. Reasonable controlled evidence suggests that wake-promoting drugs, such as modafinil in standard doses, may be effective supplemental symptomatic treatment. Concerns over side effects such as hypertension and relatively high drug costs have limited this approach, however.

### Central sleep apnoea

Although OSA is by far the commonest reason for intermittent cessation of overnight breathing, in some subjects the neural drive or effort to breathe appears impaired. This can be picked up as an incidental finding on an overnight recording with no obvious clinical consequences. In a minority, however, so-called central sleep apnoea (CSA) produces clinically significant hypoventilation overnight with sleep fragmentation and daytime consequences.

There are four typical scenarios in which nocturnal hypoventilation may be seen (Figure 4.5):

1. Loss of ventilatory drive during non-REM sleep may occur after brainstem damage or occasionally as a result of long-term opiate drugs. Very rarely, infants may be seen with 'Ondine's curse', in which breathing ceases at sleep onset, requiring long-term ventilator support.

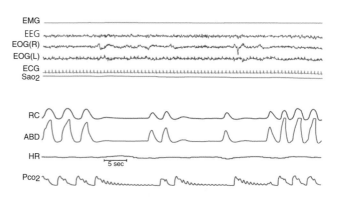

**Figure 4.5** In this example of a polysomnogram, the periodic lack of signal in the ribcage (RC) and abdominal (ABD) traces indicates a lack of respiratory effort as is seen in central sleep apnoea. In this recording a sensitive carbon dioxide ($CO_2$) sensor has picked up oscillations in the $CO_2$ partial pressures ($pCO_2$) during the apnoeic periods. This reflects small displacements of air at the nostril caused by a beating heart, proving the patency of the upper airways.
ECG, electrocardiogram; EMG, electromyogram; EOG, electro-oculogram; HR, heart rate; $SaO_2$, oxygen saturation in blood

2. Left ventricular failure can produce unstable ventilatory control ultimately due to increased left atrial pressures and prolonged circulation times. Regular waxing and waning of tidal volumes, known as Cheyne–Stokes breathing, is seen as abnormal reactivity to carbon dioxide levels.

3. At altitude, sustained hypoxia produces nocturnal hypoventilation as the hypoxic drive is diminished during sleep.

4. Weak or disadvantaged chest muscles may lead to nocturnal hypoventilation. Either neuromuscular disease affecting the diaphragm and/or truncal muscles or extreme obesity are the usual causes.

If required, treatment of CSA or nocturnal hypoventilation needs to be individualised. Non-invasive ventilation (NIV) is often appropriate. The equipment resembles a CPAP mask and pump but with pressures that vary between inspiration and expiration.

In those with heart failure and daytime hypersomnolence, the best treatment for overnight hypoventilation remains uncertain. Trials of sophisticated ventilators using servo-adaptive algorithms to 'smooth out' breathing control may show improved daytime wakefulness and increased survival in this group but strong positive evidence is awaited.

When CSA is secondary to altitude, many advocate the use of acetazolamide to create a mild metabolic acidosis that stimulates nocturnal breathing.

### Complex sleep apnoea

Some patients diagnosed and treated for OSA with CPAP therapy appear to develop CSA when subsequently investigated either as a routine follow-up or for treatment failure. This is often a transient and poorly understood phenomenon. As with pure CSA, if treatment is needed, servo-adaptive ventilators that accurately monitor the dynamic changes in breathing overnight may be used to good effect.

## Further reading

Bradley, T.D. and Phillipson E.A. (1985) Pathogenesis and pathophysiology of the obstructive sleep apnea syndrome. *Med Clin North Am*, **69**, 1169–1185.

National Institute for Health and Clinical Excellence (2008) *Continuous positive airway pressure for the treatment of obstructive sleep apnoea/hypopnoea*. National Institute for Health and Clinical Excellence (NICE), London.

Yaggi, H.K., Concato, J., Kernan, W.N. *et al.* (2005) Obstructive sleep apnea as a risk factor for stroke and death. *N Engl J Med*, **353**, 2034–2041.

Young, T., Peppard, P.E. and Gottlieb D.J. (2002) Epidemiology of obstructive sleep apnoea: a population health perspective. *Am J Respir Crit Care Med* **165**, 1217–1239.

# CHAPTER 5

# Insomnia

Dissatisfaction with overnight sleep is such a common complaint that it is often overlooked or, at best, incompletely assessed. Indeed, if specifically asked about sleep quality, approximately one-third of those visiting a general practitioner will report problems, a proportion that rises to two-thirds of those attending psychiatry services. Insomnia is reported more in females and generally increases with age.

Transient or short-term insomnia, usually triggered by a recognisable life event or stressor, is a universally recognised phenomenon. However, the underlying mechanisms or causes of chronic insomnia are often more obscure. Furthermore, the pathways for managing significant insomnia presenting to primary care are generally very poorly developed, creating frustration for patients and physicians alike.

Defining chronic insomnia as a formal sleep disorder is challenging, especially as it is a heterogeneous complaint. Broadly, subjects can report difficulty with any aspect of sleep, whether it is initiation, duration, consolidation or quality. The problem persists despite a desire to sleep normally with adequate time and opportunity for satisfactory sleep.

Most authorities would suggest an approximate benchmark of 30 minutes either trying to achieve sleep or a similar time spent awake after sleep onset as reflecting significant insomnia. The problem needs to have been present most nights of the week for over one month and, importantly, to have resulted in a degree of daytime impairment. Typical daytime symptoms include lethargy, malaise and cognitive blunting, especially in tasks involving attention or concentration. In severe cases, the problem completely dominates a subject's life such that vocational, social or school performance is severely compromised.

Importantly, insomnia is recognised as a reliable independent risk factor for developing depression and hypertension. Furthermore, numerous somatic symptoms, such as increased muscle tension, gastrointestinal upset and headache, are often intimately associated with insomnia.

Although the distinction may often be blurred, it is useful to consider insomnia either as a primary phenomenon, reflecting an intrinsic sleep disorder, or as having an extrinsic cause largely due to factors such as the environment, drugs or other medical conditions. Broadly speaking, an important clue that insomnia is a primary rather than a co-morbid phenomenon is that subjects report a complete inability to nap under any circumstances during the day, despite persistently restricted or poor quality nocturnal sleep. At its simplest, a subject with primary insomnia can be considered 'tired but wired'.

## Mechanisms of insomnia

There are at least four interacting factors that can contribute to insomnia in clinical practice.

### Homeostatic factors

It should be emphasised that normal sleepiness is a true drive state that builds exponentially with prolonged wakefulness and

*ABC of Sleep Medicine*, First Edition. Paul Reading.
© 2013 John Wiley & Sons, Ltd. Published 2013 by John Wiley & Sons, Ltd.

which can only be satiated by sleep itself. If the sleep drive is 'weak' for some reason or, perhaps more commonly, if someone is overly aroused or 'wakeful', insomnia may result. Although the neurochemistry of arousal and sleep onset systems in the brain is increasingly understood, consistent or objective abnormalities in insomniacs are difficult to demonstrate with current technology, even in severe cases. This may partly be due to the heterogeneous nature of the condition.

## Inhospitable environment

A large number of adverse environmental factors may interfere with sleep and might not be readily recognised by an insomniac (Box 5.1). Alternatively, it is not uncommon for a person to recognise a possible cause for their insomnia but be unaware that there may be a potential remedy. Successful treatment of a bed partner's severe snoring is a relatively common example.

| Box 5.1 **Common environmental causes of insomnia** | |
| --- | --- |
| Loud noises | Bed partner (snoring, coughing, sleep-talking) or pets (e.g. barking); |
| | music, television, telephone; |
| | traffic, trains, mechanical sounds (e.g. a lift) |
| Extreme temperature | Heat (no air conditioning in hot climates); |
| | cold (insufficient bedcovers or their removal during night) |
| Bedding materials | Bed or pillow uncomfortable; |
| | Allergy to washing powder or feathers in pillow |
| Light | Bright light during summer in high latitudes; |
| | Normal sunlight during the day if working night shifts |
| Body positioning | Seated position (e.g. when using public transport); |
| | Cramped bed if subject or partner significantly obese |
| Movement | Vibration or turbulence if sleeping on public transport; |
| | Body movements (e.g. leg kicks from partner) |

Up to 20% of people are aware there may be excessive noise in the sleeping environment. This may not be enough to fully wake subjects but might produce lighter and less refreshing sleep. Almost certainly, subjects vary in their ability to 'gate' extrinsic predictable noises at night, explaining why many find it possible to sleep peacefully next to train lines.

## Maladaptive coping mechanisms and behaviours

Many potentially reversible behaviours, habits or beliefs exist to promote or worsen insomnia (Box 5.2).

| Box 5.2 **Maladaptive behaviours that can compromise sleep quality** |
| --- |
| • Engaging in stimulating activities up to the point of bedtime |
| • Using the bedroom for activities other than sleep |
| • Inconsistent sleep–wake rhythm through the week |
| • Excessive checking of the clock during the night |
| • Consuming foods before bed that might promote acid reflux and heartburn |
| • Inappropriate caffeine intake |
| • Using alcohol habitually as a sleep aid |
| • Inadequate physical activity or exercise during the day |

It is obvious that both the body and mind need to be in a relaxed state before sleep can be initiated. This can often be overlooked with increasing trends for people to engage in work or other arousing activities right up to the intended time of sleep onset. The consequent inability to suddenly fall asleep then creates frustration and fuels further problems.

Insomniacs will often lose confidence that they can fall asleep in their bedrooms by a process of negative conditioning. Such patients will report significant sleepiness late evening whilst relaxing in the living room which disappears immediately they enter the bedroom. The failure of the bedroom to cue sleep occurs particularly in those who habitually use the room for activities such as studying or paying bills, for example. Paradoxically, compared to good sleepers, subjects with this type of insomnia generally spend an inordinate large amount of time in the bedroom across 24 hours but a much smaller proportion of it actually asleep (Figure 5.1).

Excessively sedentary lifestyles or very irregular sleep–wake schedules across a working week and weekend can also contribute to insomnia and not readily be recognised by the subject as provoking factors.

Awareness of the passage of time through the night and persistent checking of the time can lead to distress and increased alertness.

Responsiveness to caffeine is variable from person to person. Some may experience fragmented nocturnal sleep even with 100 mg or less taken in the morning, equivalent to a large cup of coffee.

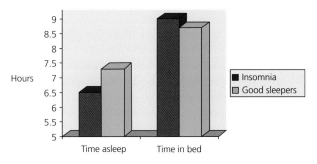

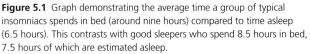

**Figure 5.1** Graph demonstrating the average time a group of typical insomniacs spends in bed (around nine hours) compared to time asleep (6.5 hours). This contrasts with good sleepers who spend 8.5 hours in bed, 7.5 hours of which are estimated asleep.

## Stress response

Attitudes and the ability to cope with normal stressors show a tremendous amount of individual variability. Recent evidence suggests that insomniacs are comparatively overreactive both to stress and potentially disruptive environmental stimuli such as extremes of temperature. This increased reactivity may be compounded by any underlying anxiety or mood disorder.

## Psychophysiological insomnia

This is by far the commonest form of chronic primary insomnia, reflecting an interaction of psychological and physical factors. Although the precise neurobiology remains obscure, underlying theories of how it develops have been well rehearsed.

At some level, the subject is considered to have an underlying, partly genetic, predisposition to developing insomnia, perhaps reflecting an ill-defined tendency for cognitive 'over-arousal'. Typically, sleep will be relatively normal until an event or medical condition triggers sleep disruption. Common examples include child birth, bereavement of a family member or an arduous shift work schedule. The ensuing preoccupation with insomnia then dominates the picture, months or years after the initial trigger has disappeared. As a result, the increased effort a subject puts into the normally automatic process of sleep initiation becomes counterproductive and actively contributes to sleep disruption. For many, intrusive ruminations and concerns over impaired performance during the subsequent working day following disrupted nocturnal sleep may further inhibit the ability to sleep.

A proportion of insomniac subjects appear to overestimate or overreact to their perceived poor sleep quality. A minority may even display so-called 'paradoxical insomnia', formerly known as sleep–wake misperception. In this, objective measures of sleep quantity and quality are within normal limits, in contrast to the subject's report or expectations.

## Managing primary insomnia

Any initial assessment of insomnia should clarify the nature, longevity and severity of the problem. This is usually not time consuming and requires only a few directed questions, primarily to rule out potentially treatable co-morbid conditions or other sleep disorders. Not uncommonly, conditions such as restless legs syndrome and 'clock' problems, such as delayed sleep phase syndrome, may masquerade as primary insomnia.

In sleep clinics, if the history is clear for primary or psychophysiological insomnia, diagnostic tests are rarely useful or required and may even be counterproductive or produce misleading data. In particular, when undergoing polysomnography, some subjects sleep particularly badly if closely monitored overnight whereas others find they sleep more easily when away from their normal bedroom environment. Wrist actigraphy (Chapter 3) is occasionally used to explore sleep–wake cycles at home over a period of weeks, particularly if there are suspicions of paradoxical insomnia.

Sleep diaries or logs can be very useful in identifying and monitoring progress in insomnia patients in whom there is poor

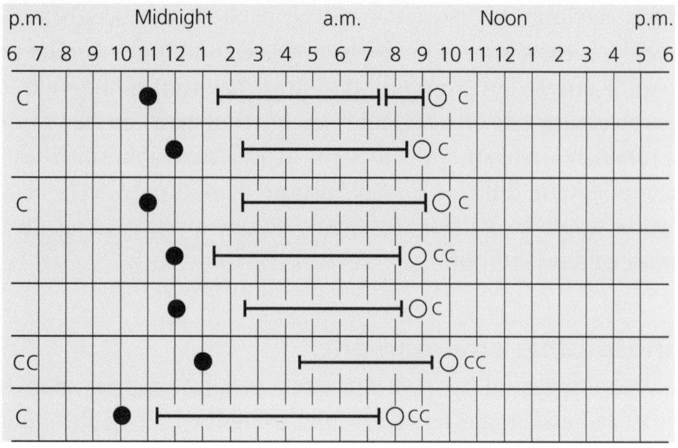

**Figure 5.2** Example of a simple self-completed sleep diary filled out prospectively over a week. Closed and open circles refer to times of going to bed and arising in the morning, respectively; the lines are the estimated sleep time; C = cup of coffee.

sleep hygiene or inappropriate scheduling (Figure 5.2). A diary should be simple, possibly using a graphical format over 24 hours. Ideally, it should show estimates of sleep and wake onset compared to time in bed as well as the timing of medication, including coffee consumption. The best information is obtained when a diary is filled out prospectively for at least two weeks.

## Sleep hygiene

A central tenet of any treatment for insomnia is the concept of good 'sleep hygiene', although relatively few patients or, indeed, physicians have a full understanding of all the factors involved. The two key elements comprise optimisation of the sleeping environment and improving routines or attitudes conducive to good sleep.

With regard to improving conditions in the bedroom, insomniacs should generally be encouraged to experiment with adaptive strategies to improve sleep continuity if they have not already done so. Although obviously 'toxic' to good sleep, problems such as excessive noise or an uncomfortable bed may be difficult to resolve, particularly if a bed partner is responsible. However, some may respond to simple measures such as ear plugs. In others, however, this may focus attention on 'internal' noises, such as breathing, and be counterproductive. The temperature of the bedroom may impede quality sleep if above 24°C or disturb sleep onset if particularly low. A dark bedroom is clearly more conducive to sleep although some find complete darkness disturbing.

Many subjects with mild chronic insomnia may respond to advice on potential maladaptive routines or attitudes that have developed before sleep onset. In general, at least 30 minutes should be devoted to 'winding down' or relaxing before attempting to sleep. Avoiding large meals, caffeinated drinks and exercise within two hours of intended sleep onset is also important. Gentle regular exercise, however, perhaps early in the evening, has been shown to improve sleep quality in middle-aged and older adults.

In those who have 'conditioned insomnia' and find the bedroom hyper-arousing, it is recommended that no more than 15 minutes should be spent trying to sleep. They may be advised to leave the bedroom and engage in an alternative relaxing or potentially boring activity, such as watching television, reading or listening to music in an adjacent room, until they are once again sleepy. Keeping any bedroom clocks from easy viewing through the night is also preferable.

A consistent sleep–wake schedule is highly recommended in those prone to insomnia. A regular waking time, seven days a week, helps to optimise circadian rhythms. Daytime naps should generally be discouraged.

## Approaches to moderate or severe insomnia

There are many long-standing or seemingly intractable insomniacs who have optimised their sleep hygiene and devoted considerable efforts to improving their sleep but remain severely symptomatic. Relaxation techniques can often be helpful if delivered in a systematic or structured way. Reading materials or audio tapes with cues designed to encourage peaceful thoughts and release muscle tension are widely available. Techniques similar to yoga, focusing on diaphragmatic breathing, for example, may also help. Others might gain more benefit from visual imagery in which the subject is instructed to conjure up tranquil scenes elaborated to encompass all the sensory domains for 15 minutes or so.

Relatively simple techniques to alter maladaptive behaviours interfering with sleep onset may be offered. For those who have excessive worry or intrusive ruminations at night, dedicating around 30 minutes in the late afternoon to list and examine concerns and stressors may diminish the energy and time spent worrying at night. Any new problems that lead to nocturnal awakenings are simply added to the 'worry list' the next day.

An alternative widely used technique involves sleep restriction (Box 5.3). Subjects are instructed to estimate sleep time the previous night and then limit their time in bed to this amount on subsequent nights until their sleep efficiency increases and they are able to increase sleeping time by small increments.

---

**Box 5.3 Sleep restriction guidelines in the treatment of primary insomnia**

- Subjects use a sleep diary for at least two weeks to estimate average total sleep time (TST)
- Time in bed (TIB) is reduced until it equals estimated TST but not less than four hours (some advocate this be done abruptly, others suggest a gradual reduction of TST over two weeks or so)
- Treating clinicians may specify a precise bedtime and arising time initially
- Patients monitor their quality and quantity of sleep each night for several weeks by estimating sleep efficiency (SE), the proportion of TIB spent asleep as a percentage
- Once SE has reached a target level for a week (between 80 and 90%, depending on subject), TIB is increased by 15–30 minutes
- The process is repeated until a goal of 7.5 hours of good quality sleep is achieved
- Excessive daytime sleepiness may be experienced initially but naps should be discouraged
- Sleep latency and time awake after sleep onset should decrease in parallel with increases in TST and SE

---

Formal cognitive behaviour therapy for insomnia (CBT-I) is held by many to be the 'gold standard' for the most severely affected patients (Box 5.4). Despite good evidence for long-term efficacy, the resources for delivering this type of therapy are generally poorly developed. CBT-I combines all the advice and approaches to insomnia previously described together with attempts at 'cognitive restructuring', typically over a course of treatment lasting six sessions. Simplistically, poor sleepers are encouraged to think and behave like good sleepers. It is emphasised that their problems are largely correctable and best perceived as a 'bad habit'. Emphasis is usually placed on how good sleepers fall asleep automatically and how any forceful effort to sleep is invariably counterproductive. CBT-I can be delivered in groups or individually, usually with a manual.

---

**Box 5.4 A typical structured six-week CBT programme for insomnia**

| | |
|---|---|
| Week 1 | detailed assessment and measurement of the insomnia problem; definition of realistic goals of treatment |
| Week 2 | education on sleep and its function with particular reference to insomnia |
| Week 3 | sleep hygiene and relaxation |
| Week 4 | scheduling a new sleep pattern |
| Week 5 | dealing with a racing mind and unhelpful thoughts |
| Week 6 | putting it all together |

---

## Pharmacological therapy

(Individual drugs used to treat insomnia are discussed more fully in Chapter 11.)

Many patients hold unrealistically high expectations that a simple drug therapy will solve their insomnia. Others may be fiercely resistant to hypnotic use which is seen as an absolute last resort.

In recent years, there has been a cultural change in attitudes to the routine use of hypnotic drugs and few areas of clinical pharmacology are more controversial, particularly for treatment periods of more than a few weeks. Fears of tolerance, physical dependence, withdrawal and other side effects, such as morning hangover, have clearly influenced both guidelines and prescribing practice. Drug expense is also a limiting factor. Many perceive the pendulum against prescribing may have swung too far and that fears of true 'addiction' are overstated. Unfortunately, there is a notable lack of positive data from long-term controlled drug trials to guide management. However, evidence that long-term use of hypnotics is necessarily harmful in all cases is also limited.

In general, if it is decided to recommend a course of hypnotic drug therapy, certain principles are worth emphasising. Firstly, realistic treatment goals and an 'exit strategy' for drug discontinuation should be established. However, overly strict protocols and limiting courses of treatment to only a few days can be counterproductive, increasing anxiety and poor sleep overall. If sleep onset is the main complaint, the lowest dose of a short-acting drug, for example Zolpidem, should be considered. If sleep maintenance is the major concern, a longer-acting agent such as Zopiclone or temazepam might be preferable.

Although many drugs used for insomnia may increase sleep continuity or total time asleep, relatively few improve actual sleep quality. Rather, the relative proportion of light non-REM (stage 2) sleep is increased, which may enhance a sense of morning 'hangover', necessitating dose reduction or a change in agent. Furthermore, some subjects misinterpret sensations of increased drowsiness on waking as a need for higher doses of hypnotics before bed.

Melatonin is available as a long-acting preparation licensed for use in primary insomnia. It is recognised as safe, especially at the extremes of age. It is unlikely to help severe insomnia, however, and is probably most effective for those who cannot switch to sleep at a conventional hour but who sleep relatively well thereafter. Such subjects may have an intrinsic abnormality of the internal 'clock' mechanism, delayed sleep phase syndrome (DSPS). Melatonin taken at a low dose of 0.5 mg or less, two or three hours before intended sleep, may be used to 'advance' the clock to a conventional hour of sleep onset.

If a particular hypnotic drug is successful, intermittent courses or having a supply at home for 'rescue' therapy can be useful. There are differing views as to whether combining hypnotics with CBT-I is a useful approach given that some will tend not to engage fully in a training package if a 'simple' drug therapy is also available.

Even in the absence of overt depressive symptoms, antidepressants, particularly tricyclics at low dose, are often used empirically as hypnotic agents. However, the evidence that commonly used antidepressants help primary insomnia is very limited. Indeed, sleep quality may be hampered, particularly if there is evidence for restless legs syndrome or periodic limb movements, as these are generally enhanced by most antidepressants. Furthermore, selective serotonin reuptake inhibitors (SSRIs) tend to cause arousal in some and rarely improve sleep parameters when formally measured.

When a mood disorder is identified, sedating antidepressant agents, such as Mirtazepine, Trazadone or Agomelatine, may be useful for any associated insomnia. Furthermore, if anxiety appears to be excessive, limited evidence suggests that pregabalin or paroxetine before bed may be helpful.

Antipsychotic drug therapies, including atypical neuroleptics, often cause drowsiness and have been used by some as surrogate hypnotic agents. There is little evidence that these drugs have a useful role in primary insomnia and side effects such as weight gain often outweigh any useful effects on sleep quality.

Antihistamines are generally sedative and available without prescription. Formal evidence that they help primary insomnia is lacking but short courses may be of help with mild sleep onset insomnia. Other 'over the counter' remedies are frequently used in the absence of good quality evidence for efficacy.

## Further reading

Espie, C.A. (2006) *Overcoming insomnia and sleep problems: a self-help guide using cognitive behavioural techniques.* Robinson, London.

Espie, C.A., Inglis, S.J., Tessier, S. and Harvey, L. (2001) The clinical effectiveness of cognitive behaviour therapy for chronic insomnia: implementation and evaluation of a sleep clinic in general medical practice. *Behav Res Ther*, **39**, 45–60.

Hauri, P. (1997) Can we mix behavioural therapy with hypnotics when treating insomniacs? *Sleep*, **20**, 1111–1118.

Morgan, K., Kucharczyk, E. and Gregory, P. (2011) Insomnia: evidence-based approaches to assessment and management. *Clin Medicine*, **11**, 278–281.

National Institute for Health and Clinical Excellence (2004) *Guidance on the use of zaleplon, zolpidem and zopiclone for the short-term management of insomnia.* Technology Appraisal Guidance 77, National Institute for Health and Clinical Excellence (NICE), London.

Wilson, S.J., Nutt, D.J., Alford, C. *et al.* (2010) British Association for Psychopharmacology consensus statement on evidence-based treatment of insomnia, parasomnias and circadian rhythm disorders. *J Psychopharmacol*, **24**, 1577–1601.

# CHAPTER 6

# Secondary (co-morbid) Insomnia

## OVERVIEW

- A variety of common general medical conditions may seriously affect overnight sleep quality but not necessarily be recognised if symptoms are predominantly nocturnal and the subject sleeps alone

- Asthma, acid reflux, prostatism and chronic generalised pain syndromes are common examples

- Restless legs syndrome (RLS) is very prevalent and has a wide spectrum of severity

- Severe RLS is often not diagnosed but represents a potentially treatable cause of both insomnia and excessive daytime sleepiness

- Epilepsy or its drug treatment may produce sleep-related symptoms and poor quality sleep, which consequently may adversely affect epilepsy control

- Several rare neurological conditions or syndromes thought to reflect pathology primarily in the thalamus are associated with intractable and severe insomnia as a major clinical feature

Although the term 'secondary insomnia' is not officially recognised by the International Classification of Sleep Disorders (ICSD-2), it has intuitive appeal and remains a useful concept in clinical practice for many. Numerous potentially reversible medical factors may disrupt both sleep onset and continuity but not necessarily be suspected as a cause of insomnia (Figure 6.1).

Secondary insomnia is particularly common in virtually all significant psychiatric and neurodegenerative conditions (Chapters 9 and 10).

A clue that subjects have disrupted sleep resulting primarily from another medical condition is the presence of significant sleepiness during the day. This is relatively rare in chronic 'primary' insomnia, in which any attempts to nap after an unrefreshing or poor night's sleep are generally unsuccessful.

The deleterious effects of increasing age on sleep quality may also interact with underlying medical problems to fuel secondary insomnia.

*ABC of Sleep Medicine*, First Edition. Paul Reading.
© 2013 John Wiley & Sons, Ltd. Published 2013 by John Wiley & Sons, Ltd.

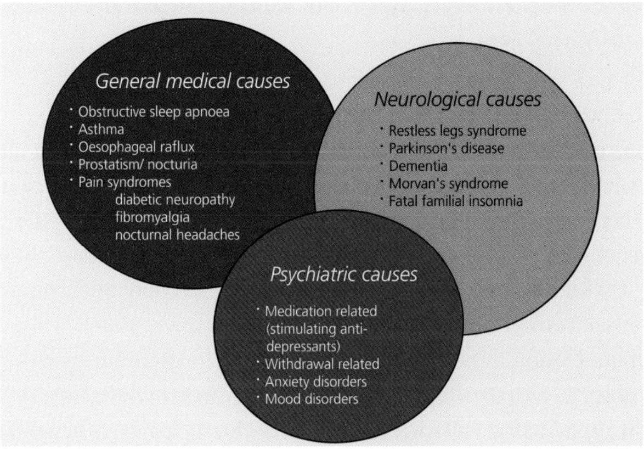

**Figure 6.1** A simple analysis of common causes of secondary (co-morbid) insomnia. An individual may clearly have more than one 'sleep toxin'.

## General medical conditions

### Asthma

In large surveys almost 50% of chronic asthmatics report waking on a nightly basis with respiratory symptoms due to their underlying asthma. It may be considered so common as not to warrant mention to clinicians. In some young patients, nocturnal coughing is the only symptom related to underlying asthma.

There appears to be a significant mortality risk associated with nocturnal asthma attacks, which are frequently an indication of an imminent exacerbation.

Peak respiratory flow measurements usually drop by 10% during the night in normal subjects. This figure rises to 50% in asthmatics due to an increased nocturnal sensitivity to broncho-constricting stimuli. Lowered plasma levels of noradrenaline during sleep, increased vagal tone and altered autonomic reactivity in REM sleep may all play a role in this phenomenon.

A worsening sleep pattern with daytime lethargy may be the presenting symptoms of worsening asthma. This should prompt extra vigilance for nocturnal symptoms and potential increases in therapy.

### Oesophageal reflux

Some subjects are particularly prone to oesophageal reflux of acid when lying flat at night. This propensity is worsened by spicy foods eaten late in the evening which may dilate the lower oesophageal sphincter. This can lead to sleep-onset insomnia in association with symptoms such as chest tightness, pain or acid regurgitation when reclined. However, the phenomenon may be unrecognised if it occurs during sleep and simply causes partial arousals and poor quality sleep.

There is also a clear association of acid reflux with obesity. In the presence of sleep-disordered breathing, it can therefore be difficult to determine the relative contributions of snoring, apnoea and acid-induced arousals.

Nocturnal coughing and laryngospasm producing inspiratory stridor can also arise from the adverse effects of acid reflux. A trial of an antacid treatment should be encouraged if there is clinical suspicion.

It is possible to measure nocturnal pH levels in the oesophagus with a probe. However, this is not widely available and remains a controversial area.

## Nocturia and prostatism

The need to pass urine at night may result directly from a sleep disorder such as obstructive sleep apnoea but can also produce severe sleep disruption in its own right. In the elderly subject, particularly if frail or suffering from mobility problems, the act of leaving the bed may produce significant anxiety and cognitive arousal, further fuelling any insomnia.

Behavioural advice to limit fluid intake in the evening is often appropriate. In selected cases it may even be worthwhile suppressing urine production with desmopressin. In elderly males with nocturia, particularly if nocturnal confusion is a feature, the provision of a convene sheath can greatly improve the situation.

Medication to improve prostatism or bladder instability in a variety of neurological conditions may also improve sleep continuity if there is significant nocturia. However, many agents used to stabilise bladder function have pharmacological actions which may worsen other sleep-related problems. For example, anticholinergic properties may adversely influence levels of dream activity and increase limb restlessness.

## Pain syndromes

Chronic pain is a common and often complex disabling symptom, affecting a wide range of subjects, both young and old. If present at night, chronic pain and the drugs used in its treatment may adversely affect both sleep quantity and quality.

There is increasing evidence from experimental and clinical populations that sleep deprivation may lower pain thresholds such that poor sleep may fuel increasing pain symptoms during the following day. This 'bi-directional' relationship between poor sleep and pain may even partly explain why some acute pain syndromes evolve into chronic pain when the original tissue damage has largely resolved.

## Neuropathic pain

Persistent neuropathic pain is a feature of several neurological conditions. Peripheral neuropathies that particularly involve the small unmyelinated nerve fibres will typically cause painful burning or tingling, especially troublesome at night. Diabetes and alcohol-related neuropathies are common examples.

Neuralgic pain tends to be more intermittent although may interfere with sleep, especially if there is a defined cause such as shingles.

Inflammatory disorders of the central nervous system, notably multiple sclerosis, are a further recognised cause of unpleasant and arousing sensory phenomena, often at night.

Although the majority of neuropathic pain agents may cause drowsiness, their effects on sleep architecture, particularly the important deep non-REM sleep stage, are variable. It is difficult to generalise but the majority of antidepressant drugs commonly used to treat pain symptoms may worsen sleep quality overall. For example, tricyclic agents often exacerbate restless legs syndrome or cause poor sleep maintenance. Neuropathic pain agents originally developed for epilepsy, such as gabapentin and pregabalin, are usually less sleep 'toxic' and may even enhance the proportion of deep sleep.

## Nocturnal headaches

A minority of severe headache syndromes may occur predominantly or even exclusively from sleep. Cluster headaches are often nocturnal, as are some forms of migraine. Both have been proposed to originate from REM sleep, occasionally linked to associated obstructions in breathing or even apnoeas. Apart from morning drowsiness, any resulting sleep deprivation caused by nocturnal headache may fuel further symptoms, especially in migraineurs.

Hypnic headache is a rare and poorly understood condition in which subjects awake with variable but severe pain symptoms at a particular time each night, usually between 1:00 and 2:00 a.m. It generally affects the elderly and anecdotally responds to caffeine or indomethacin before bed.

## Fibromyalgia

Fibromyalgia is an extremely prevalent generalised musculoskeletal pain syndrome that affects up to 2% of the population. Precise criteria for clinical diagnosis are lacking although there is often overlap with chronic fatigue syndrome. Nocturnal sleep in fibromyalgia is usually unrefreshing in the absence of pathognomonic or specific abnormalities. When formally studied, sleep maintenance is generally poor with reduced levels of deep non-REM sleep. Non-specific phenomena may also be picked up on a polysomnogram recording. For example, a lack of sleep spindles (in light sleep) and so-called 'alpha intrusions' (in deep sleep) have been described as likely indicators of poor quality nocturnal sleep.

Improving nocturnal sleep in subjects with fibromyalgia can often also improve daytime pain and quality of life measures. Exercise therapy or other alternative approaches are often more successful than drugs in this respect. However, if drug therapy is considered, agents that have the least adverse effects on overnight sleep quality are more likely to be successful.

## Neurological conditions

### Restless legs syndrome

Restless legs syndrome (RLS) is a clinical diagnosis based on responses to four key questions (Table 6.1). Most sufferers will

**Table 6.1** Diagnosis of (restless legs syndrome) RLS depends on a positive response to four key symptoms.

| Key symptoms of RLS | Comment |
| --- | --- |
| An urge to physically move the legs usually with an ill-described discomfort in the affected limb(s) | The arms or even other body parts may be involved in severe cases |
| Symptoms worse or exclusively linked to relaxing or sitting quietly | Persistence of discomfort with activity usually indicates an alternative diagnosis |
| Rubbing or moving affected limb results in temporary relief of symptoms | Symptoms return when once again rested; other strategies include applying cold or hot stimuli to the limb or hanging the leg out of the bed |
| Symptoms invariably worse or only present in the late evening or when trying to achieve sleep | Severe cases, often on drug treatment, may report symptoms early in the afternoon |

**Table 6.2** Some common associations of RLS.

| Condition associated with RLS | Comment |
| --- | --- |
| Iron deficiency | Ferritin levels should generally be checked even in the absence of anaemia; serum levels of ferritin may not correlate well with brain iron levels |
| Pregnancy | RLS very common in late pregnancy with relief after delivery of the baby |
| Renal failure | RLS is very common in chronic renal failure and often overlooked; dialysis is made particularly uncomfortable; reduced availability of iron may explain the association |
| Peripheral neuropathy | Although a controversial area, some studies have indicated subclinical neuropathy in the majority of RLS subjects |
| Depression | RLS may predispose to depression or, alternatively, be exaggerated by the majority of antidepressant drugs |
| Hypertension | Increasing evidence suggests sympathetic overactivity in RLS, with hypertension as one of the likely consequences |

describe an ill-defined ache or 'itch' under the skin around the shins or thighs that causes them to feel restless. Rubbing or moving the affected limb produces temporary relief. Symptoms are invariably worse in the evening or when trying to sleep.

RLS is most often an intermittent and trivial phenomenon affecting up to 5% of the population. At the severe end of the spectrum, however, subjects report severe insomnia and subsequent disabling daytime somnolence. Furthermore, associated leg movements during sleep (regular or 'periodic' limb jerking) may further worsen the sleep quality of severe cases as well as that of their bed partners. Active treatment is usually appropriate in those moderately or severely symptomatic on at least three evenings per week.

RLS is associated with a variety of conditions (Table 6.2) although the precise neurobiology remains obscure. There is frequently a strong familial component suggesting an autosomal dominant inheritance pattern, particularly in patients reporting symptoms before 40 years of age. Recent advances have implicated genes involved in spinal cord development as conferring particular risk for the condition.

Based on a variety of evidence, including specialised imaging, current theories suggest that brain iron deficiency may lie behind most forms of RLS. It is therefore important to screen also for peripheral deficiency of iron stores. If ferritin levels are below 50 mg/l, iron supplementation is recommended, even in the absence of frank anaemia.

Treatment options, when required, are listed in Table 6.3. The evidence base is most established for dopamine agonist therapy using doses generally much lower than those for Parkinson's disease. Side effects such as nausea may limit usefulness, as may the development of augmentation. The latter refers to worsening symptoms despite an initial response to therapy. In particular, uncomfortable restlessness extends to other part of the body, such as the arms, and occurs earlier in the day than previously. At this point, alternative treatment strategies are usually indicated, since increasing dopamine agonist drug doses further generally worsens the situation.

**Table 6.3** A summary of commonly used drugs for RLS. It should be noted that controlled evidence and formal licenses for prescribing exist only for the dopamine agonist drugs.

| Drug treatment for RLS | Comment |
| --- | --- |
| Dopamine agonists (DAs) | The commonly used non-ergot DAs (pramipexole, ropinirole and rotigotine) are all licensed for RLS and considered first-line therapy in moderate or severe cases; doses are generally lower than those used for Parkinson's disease |
| Levo-DOPA | Levo-DOPA can be effective but is best used as an intermittent therapy due to rebound symptoms and augmentation occurring with prolonged courses (see text) |
| Opiates | Codeine and more powerful opiates can be effective for symptomatic control; fears over side effects and dependence limit their use |
| Anticonvulsants | Agents such as gabapentin or pregabalin can be useful as second-line (unlicensed) medications, particularly if the sensory component is prominent |
| Sedatives or hypnotics | Agents such as clonazepam may be used to improve sleep continuity non-specifically; risks of morning 'hangover' and increased snoring may limit usefulness |

RLS usually responds to opiate medication although it is rare to recommend long-term courses or regular treatment. However, supplemental codeine or more powerful opioid agents may be useful strategies for transient worsening of RLS symptoms. A variety of agents initially developed as anti-epileptic drugs may also have a useful role in RLS. There is most evidence for pregabalin and gabapentin, particularly if the sensory component of the RLS symptomology is prominent.

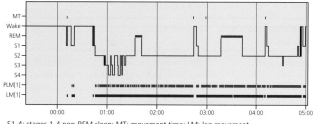

S1-4: stages 1-4 non-REM sleep; MT: movement time; LM: leg movement

**Figure 6.2** A hypnogram of a middle-aged male with severe RLS and associated periodic limb movements (PLMs). The trace shows a sleep-onset insomnia (due to RLS) and subsequent very frequent PLMs through the whole sleeping period. The PLMs were partially arousing the subject and preventing deep (stage 3 and 4) non-REM sleep.

Routine hypnotics are sometimes used as a non-specific therapy in RLS to improve sleep continuity. Clonazepam in standard doses is most commonly used although it may lead to morning drowsiness.

Controlled evidence is accumulating that courses of intravenous iron therapy may help severe and resistant RLS even if there is no evidence for peripheral iron deficiency. Symptom relief can extend for months in some cases. Specialist supervision is needed to reduce the risk of anaphylactic or allergic reactions to intravenous iron by giving test doses.

Given the symptom-based diagnosis, investigations for RLS are rarely indicated although they may reveal additional sleep pathology in drug-resistant cases. If an overnight polysomnogram is performed, however, an excess of (periodic) limb movements is usually seen, particularly in the early part of the sleep cycle, this may help to confirm the clinical diagnosis of RLS (Figure 6.2).

## Epilepsy

Sleep deprivation is a well recognised precipitant or risk factor for many forms of epilepsy. However, epilepsy itself and its treatment may also impact significantly on sleep quality.

If generalised seizures occur from sleep there is clearly sleep disruption. However, once back to sleep after a seizure, there are also subsequent changes in sleep architecture with an excess of light non-REM sleep and strikingly reduced REM sleep.

In general, epileptic patients appear to sleep less well than control populations, even if there is no evidence for nocturnal seizure activity. If electrical discharges suggesting generalised epilepsy are seen overnight with no clinical manifestations of seizures, arousals are more frequent with potential adverse consequences for daytime alertness.

The effects of anti-epileptic drugs on sleep quality are variable and often hard to predict in individuals.

An estimated one-third of epileptic patients are significantly sleepy during the day. This is often attributed to medication effects but unrecognised (subclinical) nocturnal seizure activity should always be considered as a possibility. Furthermore, it is important to exclude co-morbid common sleep disorders causing daytime somnolence such as obstructive sleep apnoea. Indeed, if present, successful treatment of OSA has reportedly improved seizure control in sleepy epileptics, potentially by reducing sleep deprivation and nocturnal hypoxaemia.

## Rare causes of severe insomnia

Given its key role in sleep initiation, it is not surprising that pathology affecting the thalamus can sometimes cause intractable and severe insomnia. For example, bilateral subcortical strokes involving the medial thalamic nuclei can produce profound sleeplessness.

Degenerative conditions with prominent thalamic involvement also have severe insomnia as a key component. The most noted example is fatal familial insomnia, an extremely rare inherited prion disease similar to Creutzfeldt–Jakob disease.

A number of rare inflammatory neurological diseases may be intimately associated with severe insomnia. Morvan's syndrome is characterised by the presence of voltage-gated potassium channel antibodies in the serum, either in the context of an autoimmune disorder or as a paraneoplastic phenomenon. These antibodies cause generalised neuromuscular hyperexcitability with cramps, muscle fasciculations and autonomic changes such as constipation. Sleep is nearly always severely disturbed with elements of REM sleep behaviour disorder and sometimes absolute insomnia. In severe cases there is a severe encephalopathic component with prominent hallucinations and confusion. Reducing antibody levels by immunosuppressant therapy or plasma exchange is usually an effective treatment strategy.

## Further reading

Barber, P., Anderson, N. and Vincent, A. (2000) Morvan's syndrome associated with voltage-gated potassium channel antibodies. *Neurology*, **54**, 771–773.

Crespel, A., Coubes, P. and Baldy-Moulinier, M. (2000) Sleep influence on seizures and epilepsy effects on sleep in partial frontal and temporal lobe seizures. *Epilepsia*, **111**, S54–59.

Culpepper, L. (2006) Secondary insomnia in the primary care setting: review of diagnosis, treatment, and management. *Curr Med Res Opin*, **22**, 1257–1268.

Lautenbacher, S., Kundermann, B. and Jurgen-Christian, K. (2006) Sleep deprivation and pain perception. *Sleep Med Rev*, **10**, 357–369.

Trenkwalder, C. and Paulus, W. (2010) Restless legs syndrome: pathophysiology, clinical presentation and management. *Nat Rev Neurol*, **6**, 337–346.

# CHAPTER 7

# The Parasomnias

## OVERVIEW

- Parasomnias are unwanted motor or sensory nocturnal phenomena that are usually categorised by the sleep stage (e.g. non-REM or REM) from which they most commonly arise

- Phenomena such as sudden body jerks at the wake–sleep transition are common as isolated events but can produce more elaborate or complex symptoms that interfere with sleep onset

- Abnormal partial arousals from the deep stages of non-REM sleep reflect the most common type of parasomnia, affecting up to 20% of children at some point in their development

- Sleepwalking, night terrors and confusional arousals from sleep probably reflect different manifestations of the same process (i.e. non-REM sleep parasomnia)

- In adults, non-REM sleep parasomnia activity may lead to antisocial or dangerous nocturnal behaviours that may be 'goal-directed' or 'instinctive' in the absence of voluntary or conscious control

- There is very little evidence to guide treatment protocols for troublesome parasomnias

- Nightmares and occasional episodes of sleep paralysis reflect the commonest forms of parasomnia occurring from REM sleep

- Prolonged motor activity during REM sleep producing dream enactment is abnormal and may indicate REM sleep behaviour disorder (RBD)

- RBD is important to recognise as it may reflect the earliest manifestation of neurodegenerative diseases such as Parkinson's disease

- Several motor phenomena at night disturb the bed partner more than the sleeping subject (e.g. bruxism, nocturnal groaning and fragmentary myoclonus)

Parasomnias are loosely defined as undesirable motor or sensory phenomena arising from sleep itself or the sleep–wake transition. The majority can be explained in terms of an abnormal or inefficient transition from one distinct brain state (i.e. wake, non-REM sleep or REM sleep) to another. Alternatively, elements of one sleep state (e.g. the bizarre or unpleasant visual imagery in REM sleep) can intrude or persist into the wakeful state.

*ABC of Sleep Medicine*, First Edition. Paul Reading.
© 2013 John Wiley & Sons, Ltd. Published 2013 by John Wiley & Sons, Ltd.

The range of possible experiences and behaviours is enormous, from simple visual images to complex and seemingly purposeful motor activities. Many parasomnias are disturbing both to the subject and bed partner, with fear responses or physical aggression as major components. However, it is not uncommon for subjects to have no subsequent recollection of their nocturnal disturbances, even if complex and prolonged. Some parasomnias are simply 'annoying' to the bed partner, with no obvious adverse consequences to the sleeping subjects themselves.

Parasomnias are generally classified according to the state of sleep from which they arise.

## Parasomnias at the wake–sleep transition

Hypnic jerks are common slightly unsettling experiences that occur just at the point of sleep onset. Likened to a sudden sensation of falling through space, an abrupt and generalised 'body twitch' occurs, occasionally in association with brief a sensory symptom such as a 'flash' or 'explosion'. Although this can cause alarm and produce a degree of sleep onset insomnia, drug treatment is rarely appropriate. Given the possible link to sleep deprivation, advice on sleep hygiene and reassurance are usually sufficient and appropriate.

A rare condition termed propriospinal myoclonus may also cause vigorous jerks whilst lying flat at the point of sleep onset. The movements tend to cause flexion of the trunk and occur on a nightly basis as the subject drifts to sleep. Insomnia may result and be difficult to treat. Occasionally a spinal cord lesion may generate these movements and spinal magnetic resonance imaging is indicated.

Often on a background of head banging or body rocking as young children, some adults may exhibit persistent rhythmical movements as they are dropping off to sleep. This may be viewed as a comforting habit or an aid to sleep onset but, surprisingly, movements also occur during deep sleep and disturb the bed partner. Typical patterns of movement include rolling of the body or slow rhythmical shaking of the head from side to side. Drug treatment is rarely helpful.

## Parasomnias from deep non-REM (slow wave) sleep

A spectrum of abnormal behaviours may occur from the deepest stages of non-REM sleep (slow wave sleep) and may affect up to

2% of adult populations. There is usually a history of parasomnia activity in childhood which can range from simple sleep talking or walking to agitated night terrors. A positive family history is also frequently seen.

As with children, this type of parasomnia is thought to reflect partial arousal from the first period of deep non-REM sleep. The subject may appear awake and have open eyes but there is little or no conscious awareness. Recollection of the disturbance the following morning is usually minimal. Behaviours are often benign but can be surprisingly complex and involve navigation through rooms or the use of familiar household objects.

Non-specific fear or agitation is a common association and may cause the subject to shout out or rapidly leave the bed. There is rarely true dream recall although a sense of a 'presence' in the room may be reported. Other common themes are visual hallucinations of spiders, for example, or simply a sense of impending doom. In this state, injurious behaviours may result in the rush to leave the room or aggression can be displayed to bed partners, particularly by male subjects.

Compared to children, during non-REM sleep parasomnias adults tend to display more instinctive behaviours that are goal-orientated. Uninvited sexual advances to a bed partner may cause marital disharmony or, at the very least, embarrassment. Similarly, nocturnal eating or cooking with no clear conscious control can be hazardous and also cause excessive weight gain. Some male subjects will regularly urinate in inappropriate places, such as cupboards.

The cause of non-REM sleep parasomnias remains obscure. Although unproven, an abnormality of neurodevelopment or maturation involving the sleep centres in the brainstem appears most plauible. Particularly in adults, factors that deepen sleep (typically sleep deprivation) or inhibit full arousal from sleep (short-acting hypnotic agents) can occasionally trigger parasomnias. Equally, factors that potentially cause partial arousals from deep sleep are often relevant. Examples include an uncomfortable sleeping environment such as a sofa, snoring or extraneous noise, a full bladder, or excessive leg movements. Anecdotally, increased stress or having an 'overactive mind' can be a relevant precipitant (Table 7.1).

The role of alcohol as a potential trigger for non-REM parasomnia activity is controversial, particularly if violent or antisocial behaviour has occurred, potentially leading to medico-legal consequences. Significant alcohol intake before bed can certainly influence the nature and quality of any subsequent sleep but no rigorous studies have addressed its specific effects on sleepwalking in those predisposed to the phenomenon. In clinical practice, some subjects report a definite link to excessive alcohol intake whereas others claim it makes them less likely to exhibit disturbances. It seems probable that the secondary effects of excessive alcohol may be particularly important as possible triggers for parasomias. For example, associated sleep deprivation, increased snoring, a full bladder or sleeping in an uncomfortable environment such as the sofa may increase the likelihood of a parasomnia occurring.

It is rare for investigations to help greatly either in the diagnosis or management of non-REM parasomnias unless there is a co-morbid sleep disorder fuelling the situation. It is not uncommon for clinicians to wrongly suspect nocturnal epilepsy as an alternative diagnosis, which may justify overnight polysomnographic

**Table 7.1** Predisposing and precipitating factors in non-REM parasomnias ('arousal disorders').

| | Important factors | Comment |
|---|---|---|
| **Predisposition for non-REM parasomnias (e.g. sleepwalking)** | Abnormal maturation of 'sleep centres' in brain during early childhood | Proposed mechanism to explain abnormal partial arousals from deep non-REM sleep |
| | The process is presumably under genetic control | There is commonly a strong family history of non-REM sleep parasomnias although the nature may vary across generations (e.g. night terrors versus benign sleepwalking); |
| | | Relevant genetic linkage studies are awaited |
| **Potential triggers or precipitants** | Deeper non-REM sleep than usual | Prior sleep deprivation or previous night shift work are common factors causing deeper non-REM sleep as a 'rebound' phenomenon |
| | | Deep non-REM sleep becomes less pronounced by early adulthood potentially explaining why many 'grow out' of sleepwalking, for example |
| | Arousals to full wakefulness inhibited | Common examples include CNS depressant drugs such as short-acting hypnotics, alcohol, major tranquilisers or lithium, often in combination |
| | Increased arousals from deep non-REM sleep | Environmental stimuli such as loud noises can be used experimentally to induce sleepwalking in predisposed adults; |
| | | Any cause of 'secondary insomnia' can potentially fuel arousals that lead to a parasomnia |
| | | Snoring and medical disorders such as oesophageal reflux may predominate in adults |
| | | In children, fevers are common triggers |
| | Psychological distress | Increased anxiety levels are often reported as a trigger although systematic evidence is lacking |

recording (Chapter 8 gives more discussion on this differential diagnosis). In a sleep laboratory, it is rare to capture parasomnia events although several sudden arousals from deep non-REM sleep to apparent wakefulness during the night, even in the absence of confusion, may act as a useful marker in those predisposed to the phenomenon (Figure 7.1).

Although parasomnias are relatively common and potentially dangerous or disturbing, there is very little evidence to guide treatment strategies. Measures such as locking windows or doors may be necessary if events are particularly agitated. Similarly, subjects are encouraged to wear bedclothes to avoid embarrassment in hotels if they are prone to sleepwalking. In general, the avoidance of sleep deprivation and assessment of any underlying sleep disorders causing sleep disruption, such as severe snoring, is

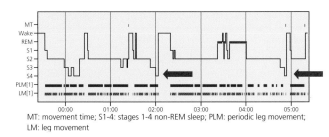

MT: movement time; S1-4: stages 1-4 non-REM sleep; PLM: periodic leg movement;
LM: leg movement

**Figure 7.1** The overnight hypnogram of a young adult subject experiencing frequent agitated parasomnias. The arrows at around 2:00 a.m. and 5:00 a.m. indicate two sudden arousals from deep (stage 4) non-REM sleep with brief apparent awakenings and associated confusion. Such arousals are commonly seen in those predisposed to non-REM sleep parasomnias such as sleepwalking.

In this case, there are very frequent periodic leg movements as seen on the PLM trace. These leg movements were important as triggers for the abnormal partial arousals that led to parasomnia activity. Drug treatment of the excessive leg movements resolved the parasomnia.

advisable. Psychological management of underlying stress may also be appropriate in certain cases.

Given the intermittent nature of parasomnias, it is rare to recommend long-term drug treatment. However, if behaviours are particularly troublesome or frequent, short courses of hypnotic agents such as clonazepam (0.25–1 mg) or melatonin (2–5 mg) before bed may be helpful. Shorter-acting drugs such as zolpidem have been reported to exacerbate the problem and should probably be avoided. Individual case reports suggest that a variety of routine antidepressant agents (e.g. paroxetine) may also reduce non-REM sleep parasomnias although the mechanism remains obscure. If nocturnal sleep eating is the main concern, some authorities recommend the anti-epileptic drug topiramate (25–50 mg nocte). This drug may work by suppressing appetite, thereby reducing the drive to eat during the seemingly automatic state of parasomnia.

## Parasomnias from REM sleep

### Nightmares

The vast majority of people have experienced occasional nightmares, especially when young. However, episodes frequent enough to cause concern probably affect up to 4% of the adult population. Underlying psychopathology, substance abuse and the use of medications such as beta-blockers may contribute. Post-traumatic stress disorder is strongly linked to recurrent unpleasant dreams related to the original traumatic event.

If necessary, the best management approach is probably psychotherapeutic, using behavioural techniques or even hypnosis. The conscious rehearsal before bed of previous unpleasant dreams engineered to have a 'happy ending' is a commonly used technique. However, a course of an agent, typically an antidepressant, to suppress REM sleep may be warranted.

### Sleep paralysis

Brief episodes of disturbing paralysis on waking from sleep may be experienced as occasional phenomena in up to 10% of adults.

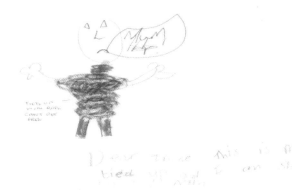

**Figure 7.2** A drawing from a six-year-old child with narcolepsy and prominent REM sleep-related nocturnal phenomena, including sleep paralysis.

Although very infrequent, the profound loss of voluntary muscle control is so frightening as to be well remembered by most, especially if there are accompanying visual or auditory hallucinatory experiences. The disturbance reflects the persistence of muscle atonia, usually seen in normal REM sleep, into the wakeful state.

In a minority of subjects, the events occur several times a month, often in clusters and occasionally at sleep onset. If necessary, a course of a tricyclic drug such as clomipramine (25 mg nocte) usually helps the situation.

Sleep paralysis in association with severe sleepiness and other REM sleep-related phenomena should raise the possibility of narcolepsy as an underlying diagnosis. This can be particularly disturbing for narcoleptic children and produce a morbid fear of going to sleep (Figure 7.2).

### REM sleep behaviour disorder

Vivid or narrative dreams are most closely associated with the REM sleep stage. In normal REM sleep only the eyes and diaphragm should move. Indeed, descending inhibitory impulses from the brainstem actively inhibit voluntary motor neurons. A subject in REM sleep is completely 'floppy' and would be areflexic if examined with a tendon hammer.

In REM sleep behaviour disorder (RBD) this mechanism can fail, causing subjects to literally 'act out' their internal dreams (Figure 7.3). This parasomnia affects middle-aged or elderly men in particular and is strongly associated with parkinsonism, even though the more obvious motor features may develop only years later. It is a potential clinical dilemma whether to inform subjects who are diagnosed with RBD in the absence of clinical parkinsonism that they are at greater risk of developing the disease.

This finding has led to great interest in RBD as a potential window for looking at early Parkinson's disease and exploring future effective neuroprotective treatments. Recent evidence suggests that the presence of RBD may eventually predict a more complex form of parkinsonism with dementia and psychosis as early features.

The main characteristics of RBD are outlined in Table 7.2. Typical behaviours include lashing out, kicking or punching, often with

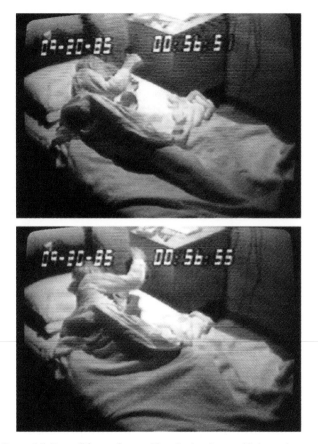

**Figure 7.3** Two still frames from a video clip showing an elderly gentleman in REM sleep vigorously acting out an aggressive dream.

**Table 7.2** Typical clinical features of REM sleep behaviour disorder (RBD).

| Feature | Comment |
| --- | --- |
| Elderly males most commonly affected, mean age at presentation is 61 | Woman may exhibit a more benign form that presents less often to the clinic |
| Movements are usually brief and explosive, involving any limb | Injuries to subject or bed partner not rare |
| Vocalisation is common | Aggressive 'sleep talking' may be the first manifestation of RBD |
| The eyes are usually shut | The subject is simply acting out an internal dream state |
| Dreams are usually aggressive or 'sporting' in nature | The dream aggression usually contrasts with a placid personality during wakefulness |
| It is rare to leave the bed in RBD | Subjects may well fall out of bed |
| Any violence is unplanned | Bed partners may be viewed as unfortunate bystanders |
| If aroused from sleep, subjects usually recall the dream they were having | This contrasts with non-REM parasomnias in which confusion on arousal is the norm |

vocalisation. The subject will generally recall the dream content if awoken during the event. Since REM sleep is usually concentrated towards the end of the night, RBD episodes are often more pronounced at this time.

The reasons why RBD affects predominantly males or why the dream behaviours are so aggressive or agitated are unclear. Increasingly, however, more benign behaviours such as laughing or singing are being described. Diagnosis is often very clear from history alone although overnight polysomnography is advocated by many to confirm the presence of abnormal muscle tone during REM sleep periods. The investigation will also help to rule out agitated or confused arousals from severe apnoeas which may mimic RBD in subjects with obstructive sleep-related breathing disorder.

RBD may also be observed in up to 30% of narcoleptic subjects although it is rarely a clinical problem in this group. Occasionally, it can also accompany non-REM parasomnias such as sleepwalking in younger subjects when the term 'overlap parasomnia' may be used. Most antidepressant drugs worsen or even induce RBD and should be discontinued if possible.

Given the nature of the problem, long-term treatment is often indicated, if only to prevent injury. There is no controlled data from drug trials but clonazepam (0.25–2 mg) before bed is considered first-line therapy by most authorities. Melatonin (2–10 mg) is increasingly used, especially if clonazepam causes confusion or sedation.

## Other parasomnias

A number of parasomnias have been described that have little obvious adverse effect on the sleeping subject but which have the potential to upset the sleep continuity of the bed partner.

### Bruxism

Intermittent clenching and grinding of the teeth during sleep may have a prevalence of up to 8% of the adult population. It does not seem to wake or arouse the subject but can lead to abnormal teeth wear and significant facial pain (Figure 7.4). There is also a strong association with migraine and general anxiety.

It can affect any age group and occur from any stage of sleep. Some view it as a non-specific marker of relatively light or poor quality sleep. It is often picked up incidentally as a 1 Hz interference pattern on the EEG trace of an overnight recording.

First-line treatment is usually a dental occlusal appliance rather than drug therapy for which there is no convincing evidence for efficacy.

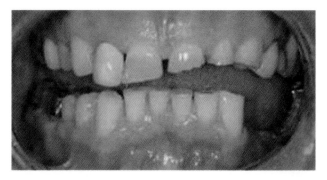

**Figure 7.4** The consequence of excessive teeth grinding in severe nocturnal bruxism.

### Catathrenia

This is a rare disorder in which subjects emit regular high-pitched monotonous groaning sounds in expiration after prolonged inspiration. It invariably upsets the bed partner and is very difficult to treat. The groans occur in clusters lasting several minutes, often in REM sleep which is otherwise normal.

It can be confused with a form of obstructive sleep apnoea or stridor but, by contrast, has no apparent adverse effects on the subjects themselves.

### Fragmentary myoclonus

Some subjects have an increased or excessive tendency for a variety of muscle twitches in the extremities or around the corner of the mouth during light sleep. This subtle phenomenon almost certainly has no major consequence to the sleeping subject and is probably best viewed as a harmless curiosity if picked up from history or investigations.

## Further reading

Olson, E.J., Boeve, B.F. and Silber, M.H. (2000) Rapid eye movement behavior disorder: demographic, clinical and laboratory findings in 93 cases. *Brain*, **123**, 331–339.

Reading, P.J. (2007) Parasomnias: the spectrum of things that go bump in the night. *Practical Neurology*; **7**, 6–15.

Thorpy, M.J. and Plazzi, G. (2010) *The parasomnias and other sleep-related movement disorders*. Cambridge University Press.

Wilson, S.J., Nutt, D.J., Alford, C. *et al.* (2010) British Association for Psychopharmacology consensus statement on evidence-based treatment of insomnia, parasomnias and circadian rhythm disorders. *J Psychopharmacol*, **24**, 1577–1601.

# CHAPTER 8

# Sleep Disorders in Children

**OVERVIEW**

- Generally, it is parents that recognise and are troubled by sleep-related symptoms rather than the children themselves
- Poor quality sleep most often leads to daytime behavioural problems rather than excessive daytime sleepiness
- Normal sleep–wake patterns change rapidly through early childhood
- Insomnia in young children usually originates from bad habits or routines around bedtime and will, therefore, respond most effectively to behavioural strategies
- Snoring is not rare in children and might indicate obstructive sleep apnoea (OSA) syndrome in severe cases, necessitating appropriate treatment, most commonly adeno-tonsillectomy
- In children, OSA can present in several ways and is closely associated with attention deficit disorder and childhood hypertension
- Persistent and excessive daytime sleepiness at any age during childhood needs to be fully assessed as it usually reflects a formal sleep disorder
- Parasomnias are extremely common in childhood and usually arise from the deepest stages of non-REM sleep within an hour of sleep onset
- Nocturnal childhood epilepsy can be distinguished from parasomnia activity in the majority of cases by history alone

## What is the problem and whose is it?

As in most areas of medicine, children cannot be viewed simply as 'little adults' when assessing and managing sleep-related problems. Firstly, with the exception of nightmares, children rarely complain of sleep disorders themselves. Whether it is excessive snoring or behavioural disturbances at night, it is almost invariably observations from parents that lead to clinical attention. Secondly, the expectations of parents may be inappropriate, especially in the context of infants' sleep patterns. A further potential issue for clinicians involved with children is that sleeplessness might directly reflect the effects of domestic stress or even abuse in a small minority of cases.

*ABC of Sleep Medicine*, First Edition. Paul Reading.
© 2013 John Wiley & Sons, Ltd. Published 2013 by John Wiley & Sons, Ltd.

With these caveats, however, it is important to stress how chronic bad quality sleep in children might well have profound adverse consequences on the developing brain, body and mind. In addition, the entire family is usually affected by a sleepless child. It is not rare for a worn, haggard parent to seek help for a child who appears ostensibly happy, active, alert and well rested.

As with adults, it is simplest to consider sleep disorders in children as reflecting either insomnia or sleeplessness; excessive or inappropriate sleepiness during the day; or abnormal activities and behaviours from sleep. As with adults, these categories are by no means necessarily mutually exclusive.

## Normal sleep in children

Normal patterns of nocturnal sleep in children are clearly heavily influenced by age.

Newborns sleep for up to 18 hours a day with alternating 2–3 hourly cycles of wakefulness and a form of 'active' sleep that most closely resembles REM sleep.

By three months of age, the sleep of most babies becomes concentrated at night with 70% sleeping through until morning. Through the first year, overall sleep requirement subsequently declines progressively such that a typical one-year old will require 13 hours.

By one year, non-REM sleep stages start to be easily identified and polysomnographic measures of sleep resemble the adult pattern. Although waking through the night remains extremely common, the important variable in practice is whether the baby quickly returns to sleep when aroused or becomes even more alert and calls out. Around 10% of parents report being routinely awoken through the night by babies at one year.

Co-sleeping with infants is common in many cultures. Potential concerns over damaging or suffocating a small baby have almost certainly been exaggerated in the past. Increasingly, in industrialised populations, it is typical for parents to sleep in separate bedrooms away from young children, predominantly to avoid the absolute need for a parent to be present at any sleep–wake transition. The appropriateness of this strategy is debated, since many parents become excessively attentive to their child when the sleeping environments are separated. Furthermore, the use of intercom units potentially fuels unnecessary parental arousal.

Afternoon scheduled naps are routine at 18 months but usually decline over the subsequent three or four years such that most five- year-olds will be continually awake through the day, typically requiring around 11 hours of sleep. Problems with sleep timing most often arise when social and educational demands are juxtaposed with sleep demands.

## The sleepless child

A systematic approach and detailed history, perhaps aided by a questionnaire, is usually helpful in identifying sleep patterns and potentially bad habits or routines. The principles of sleep hygiene in childhood are outlined in Box 8.1.

---

**Box 8.1  Principles of sleep hygiene in childhood**

- The bedroom should be dark and quiet
- Bedtime routines should be strictly enforced
- The time of morning waking should be firmly and consistently structured
- Bedroom temperatures should be kept comfortably cool (around 20°C)
- Environmental noise should be minimised; occasionally background music may help to block extraneous noise
- Children should not be hungry before bed; small snacks before bed may be allowed
- Excessive fluids before bed may interfere with sleep continuity by distending the bladder
- Children should learn to fall asleep alone
- Vigorous activity late evening should be avoided
- A bath can be stimulating for children and may need to be moved to two hours before bedtime
- Daytime naps should be developmentally appropriate and brief

---

Behavioural or conditioned factors are far commoner than any formal sleep disorder and will usually respond to a disciplined behavioural approach. In young children, the process of sleep onset needs to be 'learnt'. Establishing calming bedtime rituals or sleep onset associations is crucial, certainly in the pre-school years. Prolonged nocturnal awakenings requiring the input of a parent to restore sleep are the usual main concern. Strict protocols and adherence to programmes designed to gradually establish sleep onset associations through the night are generally successful, effectively 'extinguishing' sleep disruptive behaviours. Positively rewarding 'good' nights is also advocated by some.

A common situation arises when babies are given excessive nocturnal fluids overnight such that maladaptive behaviours and bladder distension may fuel the fragmented sleep further. Gradual discontinuation of nocturnal fluids over two weeks is usually effective.

Occasionally, unsuspected medical conditions may cause insomnia secondarily. These include nocturnal asthma, cow's milk allergy, otitis media or other painful disorders. Furthermore, the majority of neurological syndromes affecting young children will have adverse consequences for the sleep–wake cycle. This may require specialist advice regarding pharmacological treatments to aid sleep.

Children diagnosed with attention deficit hyperactivity disorder (ADHD) appear to have disproportionally disrupted sleep. Indeed, some propose that the sleep disruption in these children is the primary problem, fuelling daytime inattention and behavioural abnormalities as secondary features. In particular, as a result of poor quality sleep, children with ADHD might experience unrecognised so-called 'microsleeps'. Any sleep subsequently accumulated during the day will reduce the sleep drive at night, reinforcing the poor sleep–wake schedule. Although unproven, this speculative interpretation might explain the paradoxical success of stimulant therapy in ADHD. These drugs may eliminate daytime microsleeps, thereby improving both the deficits in attention and the integrity of the sleep–wake cycle.

A common scenario in middle childhood and early adolescence relates to inadequate limit setting, such that a child physiologically prepared for sleep simply refuses to stay in the bedroom. The ensuing struggle with parents may escalate, most often terminating with a parent acceding to the child's wishes and reinforcing the unwanted behaviour. Persistence and consistency with a bedroom ritual, perhaps enhanced by closing a door or gate to the bedroom, rather than punishment or expressions of anger are central to successful behavioural modification in this situation. Social or environmental factors, however, such as sharing a room with a sibling may complicate the issue of limit setting.

A significant proportion of adolescents might be considered 'night owls' in that they prefer to stay up late and extend their sleep period to mid-morning or later. Although behavioural or psychosocial factors may clearly fuel this tendency, it is increasingly acknowledged that the typical circadian rhythm of a teenager is delayed compared to adults such that they are, in a sense, 'programmed' to sleep and arise later.

A small minority of subjects with this tendency fulfil the criteria for delayed sleep phase syndrome (DSPS), in which the inability to arise at a conventional hour is so impaired as to cause major problems with schooling. Other than the timing, the sleep of these individuals is normal and the problem often resolves at weekends or when an early schedule is unnecessary. It is important to recognise that DSPS reflects a true disorder of circadian timing and not to dismiss the problem simply as reflecting bad habits or indiscipline. Treatments attempting to advance the clock mechanism are often justified although the evidence base is poor. Low dose melatonin (0.5 mg) taken at 9:00 p.m. may help to facilitate sleep onset around 11:00 p.m. whereas bright light or phototherapy immediately on waking, ideally around 8:00 a.m., may enhance morning arousal.

## The child that snores

Benign noisy nocturnal breathing is frequently observed in young children and should be distinguished from potentially serious conditions such as obstructive sleep apnoea (OSA) or other breathing-related disorders.

Approximately 10% of five-year-olds will snore most nights without evidence for airway obstruction or sleep fragmentation (primary snoring). However, depending on precise definitions, between 1 and 2% of children will exhibit pauses in their breathing

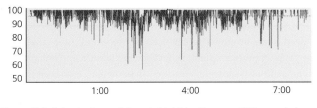

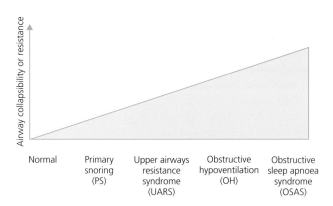

**Figure 8.1** Oximetry trace of 4 year-old child with severe OSA recorded over a night (time shown on horizontal axis). Repeated dips in oxygen saturations below 60% are seen during nocturnal sleep (vertical axis). These most likely coincide with REM sleep episodes when snoring and apnoeas are generally more pronounced because muscle tone is decreased.

**Figure 8.2** The spectrum of obstructive sleep-disordered breathing in children.

pattern, so-called hypopnoeas or apnoeas, at least five times an hour. Aside from the adverse consequences for sleep quality, secondary effects such as school failure or growth retardation can be profound.

Parents will report a variety of symptoms in children with OSA (Box 8.2). Most describe loud snoring and frequent mouth breathing at night with restlessness and enuresis affecting around 50%. Difficult daytime behaviour is also observed in 50%, with developmental delay in 20%. Overnight, children will often adopt an unusual sleeping posture with their neck hyperextended. Unlike with adults, frank daytime sleepiness is relatively rare in childhood OSA. However, in common with the adult population, increasing evidence suggests a strong correlation between the severity of sleep apnoea and hypertension, particularly systolic blood pressure.

---

**Box 8.2 Typical symptoms reported in childhood OSA**

| Symptoms at night | Symptoms during day |
| --- | --- |
| Snoring | Poor school performance |
| Witnessed pauses in breathing (apnoea) | Aggressive behaviour |
| Choking noises | Hyperactivity |
| Increased efforts to breathe | Attention deficit disorder |
| Enuresis | Morning headaches or lethargy |
| Frequent awakenings or restless sleep, often with increased nightmares | Excessive daytime sleepiness (surprisingly rare) |
| Dry mouth in morning | |
| Increased sweating | |
| Abnormal posture in sleep (typically hyperextended neck) | |

---

Although largely a clinical diagnosis, childhood OSA should be confirmed by overnight oximetry and, ideally, other measures of breathing parameters either in the home or in a hospital setting (Figure 8.1). Given the spectrum of severity of airways obstruction in children (Figure 8.2), deciding when to treat can be difficult. In the absence of clear guidelines, clinical impression is usually the main arbiter in practice.

OSA in children is most commonly treated effectively by adenotonsillectomy, which improves sleep parameters in almost 90% of cases. There is often an associated growth spurt after the operation. This presumably reflects restoration of growth hormone secretion, which occurs in the first hour of deep non-REM sleep in children. There is also evidence that school performance may be enhanced a year after successful treatment of OSA.

There may be other reasons for a narrowed airway that need addressing, such as severe obesity or a receding chin (retrognathia). The latter may reflect an underlying congenital problem such as Pierre Robin syndrome. Regarding obesity, for every unit increment of body mass index (BMI) beyond the mean, the OSA risk increases by 12% in children. A number of complex childhood syndromes may produce significant sleep-related breathing problems that may go unrecognised but require specialist treatment (Box 8.3).

---

**Box 8.3 Examples of complex syndromes in childhood associated with sleep-related breathing disorders potentially requiring specialist input**

- Achondroplasia
- Asperger's syndrome
- Arnold–Chiari malformation
- Downs syndrome
- Hirschsprung's disease
- Mucopolysaccharide storage disorders
- Pierre Robin syndrome
- Prader–Willi syndrome
- Syringomyelia

---

Rarely, snoring may be mistaken for other noisy phenomena at night, such as wheezing or stridor. The former may be limited to the nocturnal period, usually with an accompanying cough and most often indicates asthma. The latter may be seen with structural vocal cord or laryngeal pathology, potentially following any prolonged period of intubation in children. Severe acid reflux at night in children is also rare but may present as a nocturnal breathing difficulty.

## The sleepy child

If young children are observed regularly falling asleep in inappropriate situations, it usually indicates a significant sleep disorder justifying further assessment and possible treatment. Even in the absence of frank napping, daydreaming reported by teachers or increased motor activity and distractibility can all reflect manifestations of sleepiness in childhood. The most important diagnoses not to miss are breathing-related disorders such as sleep apnoea (see above) or primary central nervous system sleep disorders such as early onset narcolepsy or idiopathic hypersomnolence.

Narcolepsy most commonly starts in adolescence but is often missed and only diagnosed years later. Indeed, one-third of patients retrospectively report abnormal sleepiness that started before the age of 15. Young narcoleptics may also develop an intense fear of going to bed due to intrusive REM sleep phenomena, including sleep paralysis and vivid nightmares. This may be misinterpreted as simple night terrors. Furthermore, in childhood, cataplexy may be subtle and atypical. For example, facial grimacing and tongue protrusion is commonly seen as a response when children try and overcome focal facial weakness during emotional episodes.

Although relatively rare, conditions such as restless legs syndrome or other causes of secondary insomnia, including chronic pain, should not be overlooked as potential causes of excessive daytime sleepiness in children.

One extremely rare cause of intermittent profound sleepiness that can be seen in teenagers is Kleine–Levin syndrome. In this, subjects appear extremely somnolent for continuous periods lasting up to a fortnight. A frequent additional feature is a personality change and inappropriate behavioural responses whilst symptomatic. Overeating or hypersexuality are typical examples. Episodes typically occur every few months with a normal sleep–wake cycle in between.

Diagnosis is largely clinical and treatments remain empirical although some benefit from intermittent stimulant therapy.

## Parasomnias in children

Parasomnias arising from deep non-REM or slow wave sleep are extremely common in children, affecting up to 15% on a regular basis. These phenomena are often termed 'arousal disorders', since they usually reflect abnormal partial arousals from the first period of deep sleep. They generally occur within an hour or two of sleep onset and produce a range of behavioural phenomena from simple confusional arousals to agitated night terrors and frank sleepwalking. Adjustments to the sleeping environment to avoid injury may be justified but long-term drug treatment is rarely appropriate. Spontaneous resolution through adolescence is usually seen although persistence of the phenomenon may occur in at least 2% of the adult population.

It is not uncommon for frequent parasomnia activity to be mistaken for possible nocturnal epilepsy. Most cases can be diagnosed with confidence from a thorough history, if available (Table 8.1). In selected cases, prolonged video-polysomnography is necessary to aid differential diagnosis.

Sleep-related enuresis is usually considered abnormal if seen beyond five years of age and can divided into primary or secondary forms. The former refers to involuntary discharge of urine during sleep present continually since birth. The latter is said, somewhat arbitrarily, to occur if there has been a dry spell of at least three months and is more often linked to organic or psychological fuelling factors. Although it is often assumed that children with

**Table 8.1** Some distinguishing features of parasomnias compared to nocturnal (partial) seizures, usually arising from the frontal lobe.

| Feature from history | Parasomnias (usually arising from deep non-REM sleep) | Nocturnal epilepsy (usually focal frontal lobe seizures) | Comment |
|---|---|---|---|
| Typical age of onset | Early childhood | Adolescence | Childhood parasomnias may change with age (e.g. night terrors may evolve into benign sleepwalking behaviour) |
| Family history | Positive in around 80% cases | Less than 30% | In parasomnias, siblings or parents may report sleep talking as the only manifestation<br>A rare autosomal dominant form of nocturnal frontal lobe epilepsy has been described |
| Nature of event | Often complex but variable in nature<br>Agitation not rare | Very stereotyped events, often with focal motor disturbance (e.g. dystonia) at onset | The exact similarity of events is a very important distinction that can often be explored with videos taken in home setting<br>The precise behaviour exhibited by subject is less discriminatory |
| Offset of event | Offset usually hard to determine<br>Memory for event obscure | Offset usually very discrete with rapid return to awareness | This distinction is important and may appear counter-intuitive |
| Episodes per month | Typically 1–3 | Usually >10 | |
| Episodes per night | Usually single events, rarely 2 | Several or many | Some nocturnal epilepsies produce over 20 events per night |
| Timing | Usually within 90 minutes of sleep onset | Randomly distributed through night | This is an important distinction<br>Seizures usually arise from light non-REM sleep |
| Duration | Minutes | Seconds | |
| Triggers | Often identified | Rarely identified | In parasomnias, sleep deprivation, stress and an uncomfortable sleeping environment are often effective triggers |
| Natural history | Usually improves with age | Spontaneous remission rare | |

primary enuresis sleep more deeply than average, it is not clear whether abnormal sleep architecture or faulty control of bladder mechanisms prevail in individual cases.

A variety of behavioural techniques to modify the problem have been developed. Enuresis alarms and fluid restriction have most commonly been advocated. Spontaneous improvement of 15% of cases per year between 5 and 16 years would be expected. Important secondary causes to be considered include unsuspected urinary tract infections, polyuria due to diabetes and obstructive sleep apnoea. Enuresis is commonly seen in children with significant parasomnia activity but is very rarely an isolated symptom of nocturnal epilepsy.

Head-banging can be considered as a parasomnia at the wake–sleep transition affecting around 5% of young children. It is commoner in males and those with learning disability. It is best viewed as a comforting mechanism, partially under voluntary control, to aid sleep onset. Most commonly it resolves with age

and needs no special intervention other than adjusting the safety of the sleeping environment. Body rocking at sleep onset is a related phenomenon and similarly usually requires no treatment.

## Further reading

Ali, N.J., Pitston, D.J. and Stradling, J.R. (1993) Snoring, sleep disturbance, and behaviour in 4–5 year-olds. *Arch Dis Child*, **68**, 360–366.

Guilleminault, C., Palombini, L., Pelayo, R. *et al.* (2003) Sleepwalking and sleep terrors in prepubertal children: what triggers them? *Paediatrics*, **111**, e17–25.

Konofal, E., Lecendreux, M. and Cortese, S. (2010) Sleep and ADHD. *Sleep Med*, **11**, 652–658.

Kotagal, S., Hartse, K.M. and Walshe, J.K. (1990) Characteristics of narcolepsy in pre-teen children. *Pediatrics*, **85**, 205–209.

Sheldon, S.H., Ferber, R. and Kryger, M.H. (2005) *Principles and practice of pediatric sleep medicine.* Elsevier Saunders.

# CHAPTER 9

# Sleep in Neurodegenerative Disease

## OVERVIEW

- Sleep–wake disturbance is seen as a major component of virtually every neurodegenerative disease

- Symptoms arising from poor quality sleep and impaired daytime wakefulness may mimic those arising from the underlying neurodegenerative process

- Patients with Parkinson's disease (PD) can develop virtually any type of sleep-related symptom, often in advance of physical or motor signs of the illness

- Fragmented overnight sleep and narcoleptic levels of daytime sleepiness are relatively common in PD and increase with age

- Motor symptoms responsive to dopaminergic therapy may account for many overnight symptoms in PD

- Advanced PD with cognitive impairment is associated with very severe sleep disturbance, often with hallucinations and nocturnal confusion

- Alzheimer's disease (AD) commonly leads to disturbed circadian rhythms and sleep–wake disturbance, often with minimal insight from the patient

- Promoting daytime alertness by non-pharmacological means may improve quality of life in AD sufferers

- In motor neuron disease (MND), an early sign of diaphragmatic weakness is poor quality overnight sleep with daytime lethargy secondary to nocturnal hypoventilation

- Non-invasive ventilation is now an established and proven treatment for many MND patients with hypoventilation

Significant disturbance of the sleep–wake cycle is increasingly recognised as an integral, important and sometimes treatable element of all the common neurodegenerative disorders. The ability of carers to cope with poor or disturbed sleep in the home is often a major cause of concern, potentially leading to early institutionalised care. Many have also highlighted the inevitable rising prevalence of age-related sleep disorders as a consequence of ageing populations in developed countries.

The vast majority of neurodegenerative conditions reflect abnormal accumulation of mis-folded proteins within nerve cells, either as a pathological marker or a likely direct cause of eventual neuronal death. Preventing or slowing down this neurodegenerative process represents a future therapeutic 'holy grail'. Results from basic science at the cellular level suggest that significant sleep deprivation or chronic poor quality sleep may actually accelerate abnormal protein accumulation within cells, potentially fuelling any neurodegenerative process. As a corollary, whether improving sleep quality could be 'neuroprotective' in those with underlying neurodegeneration remains a tantalising but entirely credible speculation.

At a practical level, optimising a subject's daytime alertness in the context of a neurodegenerative illness will, at the very least, have a positive influence on attention, cognition and possibly mood. Unfortunately, many drugs used in dementia and related disorders may have the opposite effects.

## Parkinson's disease

Idiopathic Parkinson's disease (PD) is characterised primarily by rest tremor, rigidity and slowed movements with impaired gait and abnormal postural reflexes. These recognisable motor symptoms are variably responsive to dopaminergic medication, at least initially.

Numerous other non-motor symptoms affecting cognitive, neuropsychiatric and autonomic domains are now recognised in PD. These are often as debilitating as the motor aspects and frequently more difficult to manage. Their presence usually reflects more widespread neuronal death within the brain and undermines the simple notion that PD is merely due to a cerebral deficiency of dopamine.

Although initial clinical descriptions of the disease by James Parkinson himself described subjects as having 'constant sleepiness' and 'extreme exhaustion' (Box 9.1), the extensive and complex sleep-related problems in PD have only recently been characterised.

Box 9.1

Sleep becomes much disturbed; the tremulous motions of the limbs occur during sleep and augment until they awaken the patient. *[in the final stages there is]* . . . constant sleepiness with slight delirium and other marks of extreme exhaustion.

A quote from James Parkinson's original essay on the 'Shaking Palsy' written in 1817.

*ABC of Sleep Medicine*, First Edition. Paul Reading.
© 2013 John Wiley & Sons, Ltd. Published 2013 by John Wiley & Sons, Ltd.

**Table 9.1** Potential causes of impaired sleep maintenance in Parkinson's disease (PD).

| Mechanisms of insomnia in PD | Comments |
|---|---|
| Nocturnal motor symptoms | Bradykinesia, tremor, dystonia (usually early morning) |
| Primary sleep disorders | Due to PD pathology in brainstem 'sleep centres', restless legs syndrome, sleep apnoea |
| Effects of medication | All PD treatments may disturb overnight sleep |
| Depression | Often not recognised in PD, partly due to lack of facial expression |
| Abnormal circadian timing | A theoretical but credible cause of poor sleep in PD |
| Nocturia | Often reflects bladder instability and can be a major cause of concern |

**Table 9.2** Causes of excessive daytime sleepiness (EDS) in Parkinson's disease (PD).

| Mechanisms of hypersomnia in PD | Comments |
|---|---|
| Poor quality nocturnal sleep | Any cause of secondary insomnia in PD |
| Primary sleep disorder | PD pathology in 'sleep centres', sleep apnoea, periodic limb movements during sleep |
| Medication effects | Most PD drugs, especially the dopamine agonists, may cause sleepiness although mechanisms remain obscure |
| Depression | Often not recognised |
| Impaired circadian timing | A theoretical consideration |

Indeed, the complete range of sleep-related symptoms may sometimes be seen in the same patient. It is difficult to define a typical patient profile, however, and any treatments should always be individualised.

## Insomnia

Even allowing for age-related deterioration in sleep quality, an inability to stay asleep effectively is extremely common in PD. The potential causes are varied and multifactorial (Table 9.1). Nocturnal motor symptoms may predominate, especially if the subject is under-treated with dopaminergic drugs. Reported difficulties with turning in bed or limb tremor interfering with sleep continuity are particularly common complaints. Another indicator that dopaminergic medication effects are wearing off is severe pain in the latter part of the night, typically in the feet, reflecting dystonia. These various nocturnal motor and painful symptoms may respond to longer-acting drugs, particularly the dopamine agonists, taken before bed.

Fragmentation of sleep is almost certainly also secondary to the underlying disease process in PD. This is not surprising given that many areas of the brainstem, including key nuclei involved in sleep control, carry the characteristic pathological hallmark of PD, the Lewy body. Long-term hypnotic medication to improve sleep continuity may, therefore, often be justified if significant sleep maintenance insomnia is seen in PD.

Nocturia is also a major issue for many patients, particularly as they may physically struggle with mobilising to the bathroom. It probably partly reflects the increased bladder instability seen in PD, although it may also simply result from spontaneous awakenings due to the underlying disease process. Agents to suppress detrusor hyper-reflexia sometimes help although their anticholinergic properties may worsen any associated nocturnal confusion. In males, the provision of an overnight urinary sheath often improves sleep considerably.

Leg restlessness is also a common nocturnal symptom in PD. It is debatable whether this is a form of restless legs syndrome or more related to underlying PD and its treatment.

Anxiety and depression are probably extremely common in PD but can be difficult to recognise. If sleep disruption is thought to result partly from mood problems, sedating antidepressants such as trazodone or mirtazapine may help. Side effects are likely to be commoner in the PD population, however, and elderly patients, in particular, should be monitored closely.

## Excessive daytime sleepiness (EDS)

Significant daytime sleepiness is frequently seen in PD, probably affecting well over 30% of subjects. The patients themselves often appear not to recognise the extent of their excessive sleepiness, making corroborative history from a spouse or family members important. Sudden 'sleep attacks' may occur in severe cases, resembling the levels of sleepiness seen in conditions such as narcolepsy.

The causes of EDS in PD are often complex and multifactorial (Table 9.2). In some, it may largely reflect poor quality nocturnal sleep. Treatable conditions such as obstructive sleep apnoea should always be considered.

A minority of patients experience severe EDS as an idiosyncratic reaction to dopaminergic medication, particularly at low doses of the newer agonist agents. As with sleep maintenance insomnia, EDS in some subjects is likely to reflect pathological damage to the brain's sleep centres. Furthermore, disruption of circadian sleep–wake rhythms seems a likely factor in advanced disease although this remains speculative.

Once overnight sleep has been optimised, wake-promoting medication is sometimes appropriate and successful in PD. Selegiline, traditionally used to help the motor symptoms of PD, is metabolised to amphetamine and may have an alerting effect. Modafinil, the wake-promoting agent most commonly used in narcolepsy, is also beneficial in some patients at standard doses although response rates are unpredictable.

## Parasomnias and hallucinations

Disturbing nocturnal behaviours are frequently reported in PD, usually by the bed partner (Table 9.3). Violent dream enactment or REM sleep behaviour disorder (discussed in Chapter 7) affects over 30% of patients and may pre-date the development of motor symptoms by many years. Clonazepam before bed is the most

**Table 9.3** Potential causes of excessive nocturnal motor activity in Parkinson's disease (PD).

| Mechanisms of excess motor activity and behavioural problems at night | Comments |
| --- | --- |
| Motor symptoms of PD | Tremor can persist into light non-REM sleep |
| REM sleep behaviour disorder | Violent or agitated dream enactment is seen in at least 30% of subjects |
| Medication effects | Extra movements (dyskinesias) may persist during sleep due to excess dopaminergic medication |
| Nocturnal confusion | May cause abnormal arousals resembling sleepwalking |

widely used treatment although some evidence suggests melatonin may also reduce the abnormal limb movements.

Vivid dreams and nightmares can be linked to increases in dopaminergic treatment. If troublesome, it may be appropriate to reduce doses, especially if there are associated hallucinations during drowsy wakefulness.

In those with cognitive impairment or frank dementia (PD dementia or dementia with Lewy bodies), prolonged episodes of nocturnal confusion with or without hallucinatory intrusions present a difficult management problem. Leaving the bed and engaging in complex but inappropriate tasks may even mimic a form of agitated sleepwalking. Routine hypnotics often worsen the situation and exacerbate confusion. Atypical neuroleptic agents such as quetiapine or clozapine (usually under psychiatric supervision) may improve the apparent psychotic elements as may anticholinesterase inhibitors such as rivastigmine. However, these drugs have variable effects on improving sleep continuity and may worsen motor symptoms such as tremor.

## Complex parkinsonian disorders

Multiple system atrophy (MSA) is a neurodegenerative disease which may mimic the motor symptoms of PD but is less responsive to standard drug therapy. Although the pathology is different to PD, it most often produces a picture of progressive parkinsonism with prominent rigidity. Variable combinations of cerebellar and autonomic dysfunction also complicate the clinical picture.

Most likely as a consequence of widespread brainstem pathology, overnight breathing may become seriously disturbed in MSA. Vocal cord dysfunction potentially causing life-threatening stridor is the most serious consequence but obstructive and central sleep apnoeas are also very common. If overnight breathing problems are suspected, specialist intervention with overnight polysomnographic recording is recommended, especially if inspiratory stridor is reported. It has been suggested that tracheostomy may be required in such cases to prevent sudden death rather than simple positive airway pressure masks.

In MSA, dream enactment and REM sleep behaviour disorder are extremely common and may even aid with early diagnosis if

recognised. Of interest, the striking male bias for this phenomenon seen in PD appears much less obvious in MSA.

Progressive supranuclear palsy (PSP) is a rarer parkinsonian disorder with prominent gait disturbance and axial rigidity. Reduced eye movements, particularly in the vertical plane, are a pathognomonic physical sign. Sleep continuity is usually very poor in advanced patients in the absence of any specific abnormalities. When recorded, there is often a dramatic reduction in sleep spindles, the EEG marker for light non-REM sleep. Sleep-disordered breathing and dream enactment are comparatively rare, however. Technical difficulties make it difficult to measure REM sleep but severe disturbances are very likely in this patient group.

## Alzheimer's disease

Alzheimer's disease (AD) typically presents initially with short-term memory failure prior to a slow and progressive deterioration in all domains of intellectual and social functioning. The sleep–wake cycle may become significantly disturbed at any time during the course of the illness. Nocturnal insomnia, daytime sleepiness, agitated wanderings at night may occur in any combination, usually with reduced insight from the patients themselves. Significant sleep disturbances might also contribute directly to a subject's cognitive decline and, at the very least, produce considerable burden to the care-giver.

Depression may be difficult to recognise in demented patients but can present as an agitated sleep disturbance. Trials of standard anti-depressant therapy are often justifiable. Tricyclic agents should be used with extreme caution due to anti-cholinergic effects which may exacerbate confusion.

Night-time sedation is a controversial and difficult area in the management of AD. Benzodiazepines often worsen nocturnal confusion and contribute both to daytime somnolence and gait unsteadiness on waking. Agents such as low dose quetiapine may improve sleep quality without major side effects. However, there have been concerns raised over the use of neuroleptic agents in demented populations with an increased incidence of strokes seen in some studies. Anticonvulsant drugs such as sodium valproate have also been used empirically to improve behavioural dyscontrol at night, with limited success.

### Circadian problems

Reversal of the day–night rhythm is very common in AD. It may reflect Alzheimer pathology in the 'clock' region of the hypothalamus although it also results from environmental factors. Nursing homes may not provide exercise or mental stimulation during the day. Early bedtimes may also be encouraged, often simply to facilitate staff changeovers. A frequent lack of daylight exposure is also proposed as a cause of impaired circadian timing. Trials of phototherapy during the day and melatonin at night have produced variable results across AD populations but no doubt help individual patients.

The phenomenon of 'sundowning' is well recognised in AD and refers to agitated confusional episodes around early evening or dusk. There may be an underlying circadian abnormality to explain the problem. Management with drug treatment is particularly difficult.

## Intercurrent medical problems

The new development of nocturnal confusion or worsening sleepiness in a patient with dementia should raise the possibility of an intercurrent illness. Such patients are at risk of acute confusional states or delirium resulting from minor ailments such as subclinical bladder infections. Similarly, anaemia, metabolic upset or even constipation may present in unusual ways in patients unable to give clear medical histories.

## Other sleep disorders

Given their increasing prevalence with age, obstructive sleep apnoea (OSA) and restless legs syndrome (RLS) should always be considered in elderly AD patients. Indeed, successful treatment of OSA with nasal mask therapy has occasionally dramatically improved cognitive function in individual patients. Furthermore, severe OSA itself is associated with signs of cognitive impairment and reduced cortical grey matter on detailed brain imaging. Whether severe sleep deprivation, intermittent hypoxia or both are the major contributing factors is unknown. Similarly, how reversible the scan changes are with appropriate therapy remains speculative.

If excessive leg restlessness appears to fuel a demented patient's sleep, even in the absence of a clear history, a therapeutic trial of a dopaminergic drug at low dose may be justified. These agents are generally well tolerated although increased nocturnal hallucinations or worsening insomnia need to be monitored.

## Motor neuron disease

Typical cases of motor neuron disease (MND) will affect many muscle groups and progress inexorably, eventually involving respiratory muscles. Indeed, death is usually secondary to respiratory failure. In some, however, respiratory insufficiency may occur early in the disease course and develop insidiously. Because clinical examination of centre core muscles such as the diaphragm is difficult, weakness can remain unrecognised until lung function (e.g. forced vital capacity) is severely compromised.

The first signs of respiratory insufficiency often occur at night with hypoventilation and hypoxaemia when lying flat, particularly during REM sleep. Resulting disturbed or unrefreshing sleep is associated with early morning carbon dioxide retention causing headache. Daytime sleepiness is also a common consequence and usually pre-dates frank breathlessness or orthopnoea as an indicator of respiratory muscle weakness.

Nocturnal ventilation using a positive pressure mask has been shown convincingly to improve sleep continuity and quality of life in MND patients with significant diaphragmatic weakness. Survival has also been shown to improve even in patients with advanced disease. Mask tolerability and dealing with upper airways secretions are often difficult issue as patients enter a palliative phase of their illness.

## Further reading

Altena, E., Ramautar, J.R., Van Der Warf, Y.D. and Van Someren, E.J. (2010) Do sleep complaints contribute to age-related cognitive decline? *Prog Brain Res*, **185**, 181–205.

Arnulf, I., Leu, D. and Oudiette, D. (2008) Abnormal sleep and sleepiness in Parkinson's disease. *Curr Opin Neurol*, **21**, 472–477.

Bliwise, D.L., Mercaldo, N.D., Avidan, A.Y. *et al.* (2011) Sleep disturbance in dementia with Lewy bodies and Alzheimer's disease: a multicentre analysis. *Dement Geriatr Cogn Disord*, **31**, 239–246.

Boeve, B.F., Silber, M.H., Ferman, T.J. *et al.* (1998) REM sleep behavior disorder and degenerative dementia: an association likely reflecting Lewy body disease. *Neurology*, **51**, 363–370.

Radunovic, A., Annane, D., Jewitt, K. and Mustfa, N. (2009) Mechanical ventilation for amyotrophic lateral sclerosis/motor neuron disease. *Cochrane Database of Systematic Reviews* **4** (Art. No.: CD004427). doi: 10.1002/14651858.CD004427.pub2.

# CHAPTER 10

# Sleep in Psychiatric Disease

**OVERVIEW**

- Significant mental health problems nearly always interfere with sleep
- Conversely, poor quality sleep almost certainly directly contributes to many psychiatric disorders, particularly those involving low mood
- Major depression is reliably associated with an altered pattern of sleep architecture, including a short latency to REM sleep and early morning waking
- Sedative drugs used to treat anxiety and associated insomnia may lengthen sleep time but do not always improve sleep quality
- A defining symptom of post-traumatic stress syndrome (PTSD) is recurring vivid dreams, replicating the memory of the initial stressful event together with the associated negative emotion
- Sleep disorders associated with psychotic disorders such as schizophrenia are variable and poorly defined but can cause major concerns, especially if there is reversal of the sleep–wake cycle
- Antipsychotic drugs may cause significant daytime somnolence, occasionally as a result of weight gain and associated sleep-disordered breathing
- Subjects addicted to a variety of drugs whether stimulating or sedative will usually report sleep disturbance either as a direct consequence of drug misuse or when attempting to withdraw

The vast majority of psychiatric disorders co-exist with a disturbed sleep–wake cycle. Insomnia is the most closely associated problem but excessive sleepiness or even parasomnias may also be intimately linked to an underlying psychiatric condition or its drug treatment.

Increasingly, it is appreciated that the link between sleep and mental health problems, particularly those affecting mood, is 'bi-directional'. Depression and anxiety may commonly fuel poor quality sleep resulting in sleep deprivation that, in turn, promotes further mood disturbance. Moreover, reports of worsening insomnia are well recognised as an independent risk factor for either the development of major depression within the subsequent year or a clinical relapse in established depression.

## Depression

All types of insomnia are extremely common in depressed patients, particularly if they are female. Indeed, 90% of depressed subjects report unrefreshing sleep that usually arises from a combination of delayed sleep onset and impaired sleep maintenance. Waking 2–4 hours earlier than desired with an inability to fall back to sleep is also a commonly recognised pattern.

Depressed patients with insomnia usually report daytime fatigue in the absence of objective evidence for excessive sleepiness. However, in atypical depression, reflecting around 10% of all cases, frank daytime somnolence and increased appetite may replace the more typical pattern of insomnia with anorexia.

There are interesting changes in REM sleep that typically characterise the sleep architecture of depressed patients. The latency to enter REM sleep is shorter than average, a feature which may persist even with successful treatment and which is also seen in unaffected first-degree relatives. This feature has been used as predictor for a good response both to pharmacological and psychotherapeutic management. The density of REM sleep overnight is also generally increased although the initial REM sleep period is shorter than average.

It is of interest that the vast majority of routinely used antidepressant drugs are effective at supressing REM sleep. Whether this property is directly relevant to their action on mood elevation remains unclear, however.

Other recognised changes in sleep architecture, such as reduced deep non-REM (slow wave) sleep, appear less specific to depression.

Seasonal depression is seen particularly in higher latitudes. There is typically an increased need for sleep, enhanced appetite and weight gain during the winter months. Morning bright light therapy with or without selective serotonin reuptake inhibitor (SSRI) therapy is often an effective treatment strategy. There is some evidence that abnormalities of melatonin secretion, usually suppressed by light exposure, may be aetiologically important.

The inability to sleep during a manic phase of bipolar depression may present as insomnia if there is reduced insight into the underlying mood disturbance.

Antidepressants vary considerably in their sedative properties (Table 10.1). Significantly sedating agents such as mirtazapine might be considered preferential if insomnia is a major feature. The new agent agomelatine also appears to lengthen nocturnal sleep

*ABC of Sleep Medicine*, First Edition. Paul Reading.
© 2013 John Wiley & Sons, Ltd. Published 2013 by John Wiley & Sons, Ltd.

**Table 10.1** Sedative properties of selected antidepressant drugs.

| Usually sedating | Neutral | Usually stimulating |
| --- | --- | --- |
| Mirtazapine | Paroxetine | Fluoxetine |
| Trazodone | Citalopram | Sertraline |
| Amitriptyline | Escitalopram | Venlafaxine |
| Nortriptyline | | Phenelzine |

time in depression and may improve sleep quality by increasing levels of deep non-REM sleep.

## Anxiety disorders

Chronic generalised anxiety may affect at least 4% of the population. It is characterised by persistent symptoms of unease, dread or anticipation occurring on a daily basis for a period of months. Although usually considered a primary psychiatric condition, there may well be underlying medical or social reasons for anxiety which exacerbate the problem. Anxiety and associated increased muscle tension almost invariably produce insomnia, which may dominate the clinical picture.

Cognitive therapies are aimed at reducing distorted perceptions about future threats and minimising the tendency to 'catastrophise'. Together with relaxation techniques, a non-pharmacological approach often improves sleep quality as well as the underlying anxiety.

Drugs used to treat anxiety are invariably sedative. Although traditional anxiolytic agents, such as benzodiazepines, may increase sleep time, the effects on subjective sleep quality may be mixed.

Some newer agents licensed for generalised anxiety, such as pregabalin, may reduce anxiety yet improve sleep quality, potentially by directly enhancing the deep non-REM sleep elements of nocturnal sleep.

Panic disorders may present as nocturnal phenomena although symptoms are rarely exclusive to sleep. Discriminating nocturnal panic attacks from agitated arousals due to non-REM sleep parasomnia can be difficult. Because the former usually arise from light (stage 2) non-REM sleep, subjects awake quickly and often have major problems returning to sleep. By contrast, confusion and variable amnesia for the event would be expected after a non-REM sleep parasomnia which develops from deep non-REM sleep. If medication is considered appropriate, sedating antidepressant drug therapy rather than benzodiazepines may be preferable for nocturnal panic attacks although controlled evidence from trials is lacking.

Post-traumatic stress disorder (PTSD) is strongly associated with sleep-related problems, notably insomnia and nightmares arising from fragmented REM sleep (Box 10.1). The nightmares in PTSD are physiologically and emotionally arousing, typically with vivid replication of the triggering traumatic event. Treatments include supportive psychotherapy aimed at reducing arousal levels when exposed to reminders of the traumatic event. However, drug therapy may also be appropriate and recent evidence suggests prazosin, a centrally active alpha-adrenergic antagonist, as a particularly useful agent. It has been proposed that this drug may actually enhance REM sleep activity but attenuate the emotional character of the associated dream or nightmare. More commonly used drugs to promote sleep, such as benzodiazepines, paradoxically, may increase the chances of developing PTSD in some patients if given after traumatic events. It has been proposed this reflects REM sleep suppression and subsequent impaired ability to process emotional memories appropriately.

---

Box 10.1 **Features of post-traumatic stress disorder (PTSD)**

Initial exposure to an event which presented the risk of death or severe injury. An immediate response of intense fear is followed by:

One or more of:

- recurring intrusive memories of the event
- **recurring distressing dreams**
- re-experiencing the event through illusions or dissociative experiences
- intense psychological distress when exposed to factors triggering recall of the event
- physiological (autonomic) response when recalling the event

Avoidance of stimuli that serve as reminders of the event:

- avoiding thoughts
- avoiding activities
- inability to recall precise details of the trauma
- decreased ability to experience pleasure
- feeling of detachment
- **restricted range of expressed emotions**
- expecting a foreshortened future

Symptoms of increased arousal:

- **difficulty with sleep onset and maintenance**
- **irritability**
- **poor concentration**
- **hypervigilance**
- heightened startle response

Features in bold directly or indirectly reflect the impaired sleep–wake cycle associated with PTSD.

---

## Psychotic disorders

It is clear from the earliest descriptions of psychoses, notably schizophrenia, that sleep is habitually disturbed in affected individuals. However, the variable nature of psychosis and the practical difficulties associated with formal sleep investigations in psychotic subjects have severely hampered systematic studies.

When assessed with polysomnography, there appear to be no specific or diagnostic sleep abnormalities seen in schizophrenic patients. The most common features are reduced sleep efficiency and an increased latency to fall asleep (typically 60 minutes or more) although sleep time over 24 hours is often increased. Contrary to early speculations that proposed a role for abnormal dreams in the generation of psychosis, there are no consistent changes in REM sleep parameters. Some studies, however, report a short latency to achieve REM sleep, as in major depression.

Schizophrenics may have reduced levels of the deepest stages of slow wave sleep although the effects of medication may explain some of the reported changes. There is also an indication of an impaired homeostatic response sleep mechanism, such that subjects do not display typical levels of rebound sleep after deprivation.

Severe insomnia is often reported as a prodromal syndrome before a significant psychotic relapse.

In practice, one of the most troublesome sleep-related symptoms reflects the reversal of the sleep–wake cycle, such that psychotic patients sleep during the day and are aroused at night. It is not entirely clear whether this reflects a biological problem with circadian timing or simply a desire to avoid contact with people during waking hours. Very recent data may support the former explanation.

## Medication

Most antipsychotic drugs have a complex pharmacological action with varying degrees of dopamine and serotonin receptor antagonism. Older agents, such as haloperidol and chlorpromazine, have been largely replaced by atypical antipsychotics that have fewer extra-pyramidal side effects. However, even the newer drugs, such as risperidone, quetiapine and olanzapine, are associated with significant sedation that may limit dose titration. Furthermore, weight gain is a very common problem with virtually all antipsychotic drugs.

From the perspective of sleep-related problems, obstructive sleep apnoea (OSA) should always be considered if there is worsening daytime sleepiness in the context of weight gain. Unfortunately, partly due to thought disorders and delusional tendencies, many psychotic patients with significant OSA do not tolerate nasal CPAP mask therapy.

Neuroleptic drugs used to treat psychoses such as schizophrenia generally antagonise dopamine receptors as part of their action. This may cause or worsen restless legs syndrome and periodic limb movement disorder, potentially disturbing sleep continuity and increasing daytime lethargy.

## Drug dependency

### Alcohol

Most people are aware that alcohol is generally sedative at moderate or high doses and may aid sleep onset. Indeed, deep non-REM sleep may be initially enhanced by alcohol in the first hour or two of sleep. However, sleep quality is rarely improved overall and significant intake before bed can be expected to increase arousals later in the night. REM sleep is suppressed by alcohol early in the night but might 'rebound', with prominent nightmares, for example, towards morning. Furthermore, alcohol excess invariably worsens snoring and may convert simple snoring into frank obstructive sleep apnoea.

There is often a reported link between alcohol and non-REM sleep parasomnias such as sleepwalking. Evidence that alcohol may precipitate a violent parasomnia, for example, remains speculative in the absence of any appropriate published data. This remains a controversial area, particularly in forensic sleep medicine, when a court may have to decide whether any criminal behaviour was performed in an automatic state during a parasomnia or whether it was simply fuelled by the disinhibiting effects of alcohol. In many cases, it is likely that the secondary effects of late night drinking, such as sleep deprivation or a full bladder, may be important factors or precipitants for parasomnia activity in this situation.

Patients who abuse alcohol usually display a wide variety of sleep complaints, potentially covering the full gamut of disorders. Detoxification programmes need to allow for a temporary worsening of insomnia, reduced deep sleep and, in severe cases, delirium tremens. The latter phenomenon may well be due to elements of REM sleep intruding into wakefulness to cause hallucinations and agitation. This occurs because REM sleep is suppressed by chronic alcohol intake and 'rebounds' into wakefulness on sudden withdrawal.

Insomnia may persist for months after successful alcohol withdrawal and potentially precipitates a relapse if the subject attempts to 'self-medicate'. In this situation, sedating antidepressants or mood stabilising drugs are preferable to benzodiazepines, which may trigger a craving for alcohol through cross-tolerance. The use of non-benzodiazepine agonists such as zolpidem in alcoholics with a demonstrated vulnerability for addiction is also not generally recommended.

### Opioids

Sleep disruption is common in the context of both prescribed and illicit use of opioids. This class of drug generally inhibits both REM and deep non-REM sleep. Nocturnal breathing disturbances, including suppression of breathing control mechanisms, are also a potential concern. If severe, central sleep apnoea may occur and cause significant daytime sleepiness.

Those that adopt a binge pattern of opioid intake often report poor quality sleep when intoxicated but worsening insomnia when withdrawing.

If opioids are prescribed for chronic pain control, alternative agents less toxic to sleep are recommended if sleep–wake problems develop. Similarly, if there is chemical dependency, a planned or supervised detoxification programme is often necessary.

### Stimulants

A wide variety of stimulant agents, including excess caffeine, may produce excessive somnolence in withdrawal phases along with depressed mood and increased appetite. Many abusers of stimulant drug also fall into a cycle of taking additional sedatives at night to help sleep. A 5 mg tablet of dexamphetamine has the alerting properties of around six average-size cups of coffee.

Rehabilitation often requires specialist input. If caffeine use is considered excessive, intake should be tapered over a week at least, partly to avoid rebound headaches.

## Further reading

Brower, K., Aldrich, M., Robinson, E. *et al.* (2001) Insomnia, self-medication, and relapse to alcoholism. *Am J Psychiatry*, **158**, 399–404.

Ford, D. and Cooper-Patrick, L. (2001) Sleep disturbances and mood disorders: an epidemiological perspective. *Depression Anxiety*, **14**, 3–6.

Hauri, P., Friedman, M. and Ravaris, C. (1989) Sleep in patients with spontaneous panic attacks. *Sleep*, **12**, 323–337.

Maixner, S., Tandon, R., Eiser, A. *et al.* (1988) Effects of antipsychotic treatment on polysomnographic measures in schizophrenia: a replication and extension study. *Am J Psychiatry*, **155**, 1600–1602.

Raskind, M., Peskind, E., Kanter, E. *et al.* (2003) Reduction of nightmares and other PTSD symptoms in combat veterans by prazosin: a placebo-controllled study. *Am J Psychiatry*, **160**, 371–373.

Rodin, J., McAvay, G. and Timko, C. (1988) A longitudinal study of depressed mood and sleep disturbances in elderly adults. *J Gerontol Psychol Sci*, **43**, 45–53.

Wulff, K., Dijk, D.J., Middleton, B. *et al.* (2012) Sleep and circadian rhythm disturbance in schizophrenia. *Br J Psychiatry*, **200** (4), 308–316.

# CHAPTER 11

# Drugs Used in Sleep Medicine

**OVERVIEW**

- Many classes of drug, whether prescribed or recreational, are taken with the specific aim of influencing the sleep-wake cycle
- The formal evidence base for the pharmacological treatment of the majority of sleep disorders is very limited and many drugs are used empirically
- Caffeine, modafinil and amphetamine-like agents are the most commonly used agents for promoting wakefulness, often in combination
- Clear protocols for the drug treatment of chronic insomnia are lacking and long-term courses of hypnotic agents are generally discouraged through fears of dependence and tolerance
- If an agent is used to aid sleep, its pharmacokinetic profile should be appropriately matched for the type of insomnia
- Many drugs such as benzodiazepines and the majority of anti-depressants will produce drowsiness but often fail to improve the quality of any sleep obtained
- It is relatively rare for hypnotic or sedative drugs to increase or enhance the deeper stages of non-REM (slow wave) sleep

Whether obtained by a prescription, over the counter or illegally, one of the commonest reasons for a person to take a drug is to influence the sleep–wake cycle. Typically, the elderly seek agents to improve their nocturnal sleep whereas younger age groups want to stay more awake.

Unfortunately, the evidence base for pharmacological treatment of the vast majority of sleep disorders remains sparse. As a result, drugs are often chosen either empirically or from anecdotal evidence and personal experience. Furthermore, given that most trial data are generated from short-term studies, little guidance exists on the appropriate length of treatment courses.

Only a minority of drugs are formally licensed for a sleep-related indication. In addition, because sleep medicine remains a relatively new discipline, familiarity with many of these agents is low. A further reason for reduced confidence in prescribing drugs for sleep disorders is that many general physicians might feel that a certain sleep-related symptom reflects lifestyle choices more than a purely medical problem.

## Agents to promote wakefulness

The vast majority of subjects with a significant primary sleep disorder such as narcolepsy will benefit from drug therapy to improve alertness. In some other clinical situations where daytime somnolence remains severe despite first-line therapy, it may also be appropriate to recommend wake-promoting agents. The use of traditional psychostimulant drugs such as amphetamine has declined largely through concerns over dependency and the relatively non-specific mode of action.

The earliest treatments for narcolepsy when it was first described by French neuropsychiatrists in the late nineteenth century almost certainly would have kept subjects awake (Figure 11.1).

### Caffeine

Caffeine is clearly widely available in a vast variety of drinks and also tablet form. However, it can often be difficult to judge precise doses consumed; these typically vary between 50 and 200 mg. The main relevant pharmacological action of caffeine is to inhibit

# Rx for Narcolepsy

amyl nitrite

apomorphine

picrotoxin

strychnine

caffeine

baths in the Seine

**Figure 11.1** A 'recipe' outlining a treatment plan for narcolepsy described by Dr Gelineau, a Parisian neuropsychiatrist who first devised the term 'narcolepsy'.

*ABC of Sleep Medicine*, First Edition. Paul Reading.
© 2013 John Wiley & Sons, Ltd. Published 2013 by John Wiley & Sons, Ltd.

adenosine (A1) receptors in the basal forebrain. This is thought to oppose the natural sleep drive, which arises partly from increasing adenosine levels in the brain after prolonged wakefulness. There is a wide variation between individuals both in the alerting response to caffeine and the likelihood of adverse effects such as insomnia.

Although a relatively mild wake-promoting agent for most, caffeine is probably under-used as a supplement in sleep disorders that cause significant somnolence. At the very least, it can usefully improve vigilance in sleep-deprived subjects.

## Modafinil

Modafinil was first introduced as a unique wake-promoting drug in the 1980s after the serendipitous discovery that it kept cats awake for prolonged periods in experimental drug studies assessing depression. The new drug was noted to have a different chemical structure to traditional psychostimulant agents such as amphetamine (Figure 11.2). Its precise mode of action remains unclear although it appears to activate the 'wake' nuclei in the hypothalamus fairly specifically. Unlike amphetamine, it does not produce euphoria. Furthermore, tolerance after prolonged use is usually minimal. The half-life is quite long (10–15 hours) such that typical doses (100 or 200 mg) are taken shortly after awakening and at lunchtime to avoid insomnia at night.

Although modafinil is formally licensed in many countries only for the treatment of primary sleep disorders such as narcolepsy, many clinicians recommend its use in other situations. Excessive sleepiness associated with head injuries or other neurological disorders often benefit from the drug, as do patients with severe obstructive sleep apnoea who remain sleepy despite optimal therapy with a positive airways pressure mask. Furthermore, it is occasionally appropriate to prescribe the drug before a night shift at work if other countermeasures to improve drowsiness have failed.

Some claim that modafinil is effective as a cognitive enhancer or 'smart drug'. Although it remains unclear whether it improves attention and performance in those who are not sleepy, it is sometimes misused in student populations, for example, in attempts to boost academic achievement.

The more common side effects of modafinil include headache and gastrointestinal upset. It does not have the same stimulatory effects on the cardiovascular system as more traditional stimulants but blood pressure can rise slightly and should be monitored. Woman of child-bearing age should be told that modafinil is known to induce liver enzymes and has the potential of rendering standard oral contraceptive therapy ineffective.

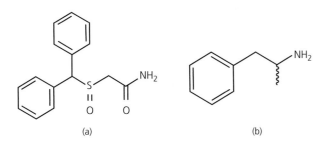

**Figure 11.2** Chemical structures of (a) modafinil and (b) amphetamine.

## Amphetamine and related drugs

Amphetamines and drugs such as methylphenidate have a very similar mode of action and are generally only used as second-line agents in primary sleep disorders causing hypersomnolence. Amphetamine is most commonly used as a supplement to modafinil or as an alternative if there are side effects. It is given in low doses (typically 5 mg up to five times a day) and usually taken flexibly. A single dose typically gives up to two hours of increased alertness at levels roughly equivalent to the wake-promoting effects of drinking around six cups of coffee.

At low doses, amphetamine and similar drugs promote the release of dopamine and noradrenaline from nerve terminals and inhibit their reuptake. As a result, the pharmacological effects are not limited to increased wakefulness. Agitation or palpitations may occur as unwanted side effects.

Amphetamine will generally suppress appetite and worsen hypertension, which may also limit its usefulness. The euphoric effects seem less pronounced when used in conditions such as narcolepsy. Indeed, frank abuse in very rarely seen in this clinical population.

## Selegiline

Selegiline was first introduced in the 1950s as a dog food additive to give pets a 'boost'. It is metabolised in the liver to amphetamine, making it useful as a mild psychostimulant in addition to its more familiar role as an agent to improve the motor symptoms of Parkinson's disease. Although not licensed as a wake-promoting drug, it is sometimes recommended as an alternative to amphetamine in elderly patients or those not suitable for more powerful drugs. Doses higher than those used in Parkinson's disease (more than 20 mg daily) seem to be safe in narcoleptics, for example.

## Mazindol

Mazindol was first developed as an appetite suppressant but found early promise as a psychostimulant in narcoleptic patients. It's mode of action remains obscure although the clinical effects resemble those of amphetamine. It is sometimes used as an unlicensed alternative agent for narcolepsy with cataplexy in those resistant or intolerant to conventional therapy.

Side effects include nausea and agitation. Concerns over a possible theoretical risk of pulmonary hypertension with long-term use have necessitated specialist use only.

## Agents to induce or improve nocturnal sleep

### General principles

Although hypnotics are amongst the most commonly used class of drugs, prescribing guidelines and protocols are poorly developed. In the last decade there has been increasing reluctance to recommend hypnotics, largely through fears of dependence, tolerance and morning side effects. In patients with severe and chronic symptoms, the poor availability of behavioural or other non-pharmacological therapies, leads to understandable frustration and anxiety, potentially fuelling worsening insomnia and an increased demand for a pharmacological approach.

**Table 11.1** Properties of commonly used hypnotic agents.

| Drug | Usual dose | Rapid onset | Elimination half-life (h) | Daytime (hangover) effects | Safety |
|---|---|---|---|---|---|
| Zopiclone | 7.5 mg | + | 3.5–6 | ?Yes | ✓ |
| Zolpidem | 10 mg | ++ | 1.5–3 | No | ✓ |
| Zaleplon* | 10 mg | ++ | 1–2 | No | ✓ |
| Temazepam | 20 mg | | 5–12 | ?Yes | ✓ |
| Loprazolam | 1 mg | | 5–13 | ?Yes | ✓ |
| Lormetazepam | 1 mg | + | 8–10 | ?Yes | ✓ |
| Nitrazepam | 5-10 mg | + | 20–48 | Yes | ✓ |
| Lorazepam | 0.5-1 mg | + | 10–20 | Yes | ✓ |
| Diazepam | 5-10 mg | + | 20–60 | Yes | ✓ |
| Oxazepam | 15-30 mg | | 5–20 | Yes | ✓ |
| Alprazolam | 0.5 mg | + | 9–20 | Yes | ✓ |
| Clonazepam | 0.5-1 mg | + | 18–50 | Yes | ✓ |
| Chloral hydrate | 0.7–1 g | + | 8–12 | ?Yes | X |
| Chlormethiazole | 192 mg | + | 4–8 | ?Yes | X |
| Barbiturates | Varies | + | varies | Yes | X |

*can be taken during the night, until five hours before needing to drive etc.

Many patients with chronic insomnia have tried numerous strategies before seeking medical help. Antihistamines available over-the-counter or herbal remedies such as lavender are rarely of major benefit. Similarly, for obvious reasons, excess alcohol should be discouraged if used primarily as an aid to achieve sleep onset.

Wherever possible, a treatable cause for insomnia should be addressed. Restless legs syndrome causing significant sleep onset problems and obstructive sleep apnoea producing unrefreshing sleep are common examples of missed diagnoses.

If hypnotic drug therapy is considered appropriate, the nature of the insomnia should be determined. A drug's absorption and elimination properties should match the profile of insomnia. Short-acting drugs should be reserved for problems actually falling asleep and longer-acting agents if sleep interruption late in the night is the major concern (Table 11.1).

Although many hypnotics may extend total sleep time, they vary in their ability to produce good quality sleep. Awakening unrefreshed from sleep is particularly associated with drugs that inhibit the deep non-REM (slow wave) stage. Finding an effective hypnotic agent for an individual may take several attempts and many subjects remain disillusioned that they cannot find an ideal drug.

## Benzodiazepines

In the 1970s and 1980s, benzodiazepines (BZs) largely replaced barbiturates as the most commonly used class of hypnotic drug. There are numerous types of BZ with varying pharmacokinetic properties although all modulate the inhibitory neurotransmitter gamma-aminobutyric acid (GABA). Because they indirectly enhance the effects of the brain's endogenous GABA, the risks of respiratory depression and excessive sedation are limited, making them relatively safe in overdose. However, if taken with other drugs that more directly affect the GABA-A receptor, such as alcohol, problems may well arise.

Potentially as a result of their anxiolytic properties, BZs may improve sleep subjectively with little objective change in sleep parameters measured by polysomnography.

The general inhibitory effects of BZs may produce muscle relaxation, memory impairment and gait disturbances. These effects are undesirable for those that need to get up through the night for child care purposes or micturition, for example. Snoring and sleep apnoea are also enhanced, especially in the presence of alcohol.

BZs are probably best used as intermittent therapy. It is important to instruct patients that rebound insomnia may be expected on discontinuation and that doses should ideally be tapered when withdrawing.

## Benzodiazepine receptor agonist drugs ('z-drugs')

Shorter-acting hypnotic drugs were developed primarily to avoid the 'hangover' effects of BZs. The three generally available 'z-drugs' are zopiclone, zolpidem and zaleplon. These drugs have been shown to be generally effective in sleep-onset insomnia with little evidence for physical dependence, even in trials lasting 12 months. Their mode of action is also via indirect enhancement of GABA function.

Although some maintain that the shorter-acting drugs zolpidem and zaleplon come close to the ideal hypnotic, confusional arousals early in the night may occur and lead to potentially dangerous behaviours. Care should be taken particularly if there is a recent or past childhood history of parasomnia activity.

If sleep maintenance insomnia is the primary symptom, some subjects benefit from zolpidem or zaleplon taken through the night if they do not have to be awake for the next four hours.

## Melatonin

Melatonin is produced naturally in the pineal gland and is best viewed as a natural hormone that facilitates sleep onset. Its release in the brain is maximal around dusk and is under tight circadian control. The robust diurnal pattern of melatonin release appears to diminish markedly with increasing age.

When used pharmacologically, melatonin can act to 'advance' a subject's clock at low doses (typically 0.5 mg or less) or to generally improve sleep quality at higher doses (2–10 mg). The former use can help jet lag or those with an extreme 'night owl' tendency. Timing is very important and the drug should be taken around 2–3 hours before desired sleep onset.

More commonly, melatonin is used as a simple hypnotic. It appears generally very safe with few adverse effects although it may lack potency. It is used particularly in very young or elderly populations although controlled evidence for efficacy is lacking. Prolonged-release preparations of melatonin have gained a licence for insomnia in the elderly in many countries although availability varies considerably. In some areas, melatonin is routinely used as a nutritional supplement bought 'over the counter', despite concerns over quality control and accurate dosing.

## Other hypnotic drugs

In the past, a variety of agents, such as chloral hydrate and chlormethiazole, have been used as powerful hypnotic agents.

**Table 11.2** Possible adverse consequences of commonly used classes of drug on the sleep–wake cycle.

| Class of drug | Potential side effect on the sleep–wake cycle |
|---|---|
| Benzodiazepines and other hypnotics | Although total sleep time may be enhanced, proportionally more light sleep is usually obtained potentially leading to unrefreshing nocturnal sleep and daytime somnolence |
| | Enhanced snoring or even sleep apnoea may be observed |
| | Evidence from case reports suggest that short-acting hypnotics such as zolpidem may trigger unwelcome parasomnia activity in those predisposed |
| Antidepressants | It is often difficult to predict whether an antidepressant drug (ADD) will be relatively alerting or sedative to an individual patient |
| | The majority of ADDs will tend to suppress REM sleep and, therefore, reduce dreams and nightmares if excessive. However, some ADDs (notably venlafaxine and mirtazapine) have the potential for suppressing certain elements of REM sleep, such as muscle paralysis, and may, therefore, induce or exacerbate REM sleep behaviour disorder |
| | Most ADDs have the capacity for worsening restless legs syndrome and associated periodic limb movements during sleep |
| | Even strongly sedative ADDs rarely produce sleep that is particularly refreshing to the subject |
| Dopamine blocking agents | The majority of antipsychotic agents (neuroleptics) will be sedative and have the capacity of inducing weight gain (increased risk of obstructive sleep apnoea) |
| | Antipsychotics and many anti-emetic drugs will worsen restless legs syndrome |
| Analgesics | Some subjects appear particularly sensitive to the effects of opiates on overnight breathing control such that central sleep apnoea may be induced. This may mimic obstructive sleep apnoea (OSA) on investigations but not be controlled by standard OSA therapies such as positive ventilations masks or mandibular advancement |
| Anti-epilepsy drugs | Anti-epilepsy drugs (AEDs) have variable effects on sleep architecture although most are generally sedative |
| | Gabapentin and pregabalin tend to increase deep or slow wave sleep and may possibly improve sleep quality if it is generally disturbed or if anxiety is present |
| | Lamotrigine is usually arousing although inter-individual differences are considerable |

Concerns over safety and dependence have dramatically reduced prescribing levels.

Sodium oxybate is a new drug licensed for use in narcolepsy (Chapter 3) which acts as an extremely effective hypnotic. It is short acting and enhances deep non-REM sleep as its main pharmacological action. It is the sodium salt of gamma hydroxybutyrate (GHB), a drug misused notoriously as a 'date rape' agent. Largely due to expense and concerns over abuse, sodium oxybate is unlikely to be used for simple or primary insomnia in the foreseeable future.

## Antidepressants

It is common practice to prescribe antidepressant drugs as a surrogate treatment for insomnia, even in the absence of frank depressive symptomology. The various classes of antidepressants vary in their sedative properties and effects on sleep architecture (Chapter 10).

The tendency for most antidepressants to suppress REM sleep has led to their routine use in treating REM sleep-related phenomena. Frequent episodes of REM sleep paralysis or cataplexy often respond well to tricyclic preparations or venlafaxine, for example.

## Analgesics including anti-epileptic agents

Nocturnal pain due to a variety of causes is a significant factor in many subjects with insomnia. Poor quality sleep has also been shown to reduce pain thresholds and may therefore promote hyperalgesia. Improving sleep in patients with generalised pain syndromes such as fibromyalgia may indirectly help with pain control.

Although many agents used for neuropathic pain are sedative, relatively few improve sleep quality or continuity. Tricyclic antidepressants often worsen any tendency for restless legs syndrome and rarely produce refreshing sleep. Opiates are also not generally effective at improving the depth of sleep and can lead to significant breathing disorders, such as central sleep apnoea (Chapter 4).

Some of the agents initially developed as anti-epileptics are effective both in treating neuropathic pain and enhancing deep non-REM sleep. When sleep patterns have been assessed in drug trials for pain syndromes, pregabalin and gabapentin appear particularly helpful.

## Potential sleep-related side effects of commonly used drugs

It is often difficult to predict how an individual drug prescribed as a treatment for a medical or psychiatric condition will affect a subject's sleep–wake cycle. Clearly, drugs that adversely affect the quantity or quality of overnight sleep might produce symptoms both of insomnia and/or daytime somnolence. Some potentially unrecognised consequences of commonly used classes of drugs are outlined in Table 11.2.

## Further reading

Artigas, F., Nutt, D. and Shelton, R. (2002) Mechanism of action of antidepressants. *Psychpharmcol Bull*, **36**, 123–132.

Brown, M.A. and Guilleminault, C. (2011) A review of sodium oxybate and baclofen in the treatment of sleep disorders. *Curr Pharm Des*, **17**, 1430–1435.

Buscemi, N., Vandermeer, B., Friesen, C. *et al.* (2007) The efficacy and safety of drug treatments for chronic insomnia in adults: a meta-analysis of RCTs. *J Gen Intern Med*, **22**, 1335–1350.

Mitler, M.M. and Hajdukovic, R. (1991) Relative efficacy of drugs for the treatment of sleepiness in narcolepsy. *Sleep*, **14**, 218–220.

Srinivasan, V., Brzezinski, A., Pandi-Perumal S.R. *et al.* (2011) Melatonin agonists in primary insomnia and depression-associated insomnia: are they superior to sedative-hypnotics? *Prog Neuropsychopharmacol Biol Psychiatry*, **35**, 913–923.

Tzellos, T.G., Toulis, K.A., Goulis, D.G. *et al.* (2010) Gabapentin and pregabalin in the treatment of fibromyalgia: a systematic review and a meta-analysis. *J Clin Pharm Ther*, **35**, 639–656.

# Index

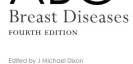
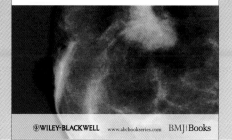

## ABC of Breast Diseases

### 4TH EDITION

**J. Michael Dixon**
Western General Hospital, Edinburgh, UK

Breast diseases are common and often encountered by health professionals in primary care. While the incidence of breast cancer is increasing, earlier detection and improved treatments are helping to reduce breast cancer mortality. The *ABC of Breast Diseases, 4th Edition*:

- Provides comprehensive guidance to the assessment of symptoms, how to manage common breast conditions and guidelines on referral
- Covers congenital problems, breast infection and mastalgia, before addressing the epidemiology, prevention, screening and diagnosis of breast cancer and outlines the treatment and management options for breast cancer within different groups
- Includes new chapters on the genetics, prevention, management of high risk women and the psychological aspects of breast diseases
- Is ideal for GPs, family physicians, practice nurses and breast care nurses as well as for surgeons and oncologists both in training and recently qualified as well as medical students

AUGUST 2012 | 9781444337969 | 168 PAGES | £27.99/US$46.95/€35.90/AU$52.95

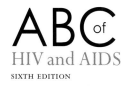
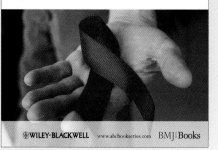

## ABC of HIV and AIDS

### 6TH EDITION

**Michael W. Adler, Simon G. Edwards, Robert F. Miller, Gulshan Sethi & Ian Williams**
University College London Medical School; Mortimer Market Centre, London; University College London; St Thomas' Hospital, London Medical School; University College London Medical School

Since the previous edition, big advances have been made in treatment, knowledge of the disease and epidemiology. The problem of AIDS in developing countries has become a major political and humanitarian issue.

- Edited by the Director of the Department for Sexually Transmitted Diseases, *ABC of HIV and AIDS, 6th Edition* is an authoritative guide to the epidemiology, incidence, and most up to date management of HIV and AIDS
- Reflects the constantly changing knowledge of the disease and its manifestations, new developments in drug and non-drug management, sociological and political issues
- Includes 6 new chapters on conditions associated with AIDS and further concentration on the community effects of the disease, and the situation of women with AIDS
- Ideal for all levels of health care workers caring for HIV and AIDS patients

JUNE 2012 | 9781405157001 | 144 PAGES | £24.99/US$49.95/€32.90/AU$47.95

# ABC of Pain

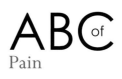

**Lesley A. Colvin & Marie Fallon**
Western General Hospital, Edinburgh; University of Edinburgh

Pain is a common presentation and this brand new title focuses on the pain management issues most often encountered in primary care. *ABC of Pain*:

- Covers all the chronic pain presentations in primary care right through to tertiary and palliative care and includes guidance on pain management in special groups such as pregnancy, children, the elderly and the terminally ill
- Includes new findings on the effectiveness of interventions and the progression to acute pain and appropriate pharmacological management
- Features pain assessment, epidemiology and the evidence base in a truly comprehensive reference
- Provides a global perspective with an international list of expert contributors

JUNE 2012 | 9781405176217 | 128 PAGES | £24.99/US$44.95/€32.90/AU$47.95

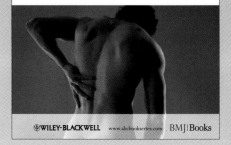

# ABC of Urology

## 3RD EDITION

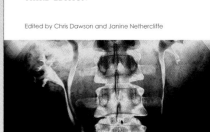

**Chris Dawson & Janine Nethercliffe**
Fitzwilliam Hospital, Peterborough; Edith Cavell Hospital, Peterborough

Urological conditions are common, accounting for up to one third of all surgical admissions to hospital. Outside of hospital care urological problems are a common reason for patients needing to see their GP.

- *ABC of Urology, 3rd Edition* provides a comprehensive overview of urology
- Focuses on the diagnosis and management of the most common urological conditions
- Features 4 additional chapters: improved coverage of renal and testis cancer in separate chapters and new chapters on management of haematuria, laparoscopy, trauma and new urological advances
- Ideal for GPs and trainee GPs, and is useful for junior doctors undergoing surgical training, while medical students and nurses undertaking a urological placement as part of their training programme will find this edition indispensable

MARCH 2012 | 9780470657171 | 88 PAGES | £23.99/US$37.95/€30.90/AU$47.95

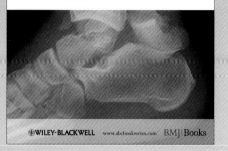
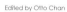
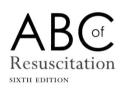
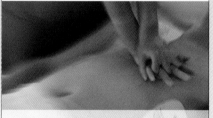

# ABC of Ear, Nose and Throat

## 6TH EDITION

**Harold S. Ludman & Patrick Bradley**
King's College Hospital, London; Queen's Medical Centre, University of Nottingham

This new edition of the established text:

- Provides symptomatic coverage of the most common ear, nose and throat presentations
- Includes additional chapters on tinnitus, nasal discharge, nasal obstruction, facial plastic surgery and airway obstruction and stridor to reflect recent changes in the practice of otolaryngology and new content on thyroid disease, head and neck cancer, rhinoplasty, cosmetic and therapeutic scar
- Has been restructured on a symptom based classification for quick reference
- Incorporates guidance on assessment, treatment and management, and when to refer patients

NOVEMBER 2012 | 9780470671351 | 168 PAGES | £28.99/US$47.95/€37.90/AU$54.95

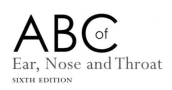
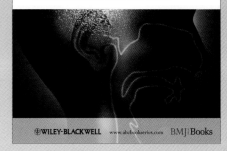

# ABC of Major Trauma

## 4TH EDITION

**David Skinner & Peter Driscoll**
John Radcliffe Hospital, Oxford; Hope Hospital, Salford

Prehospital care is a growing area in medicine, and emergency treatments are becoming more sophisticated as the potential to save lives grow. This practical book:

- Is a comprehensive guide to the management of the multiply injured patient during the initial hours after injury
- Includes new chapters on major incidents and nuclear and biological emergencies
- Provides clear and concise guidance with accompanying photographs and diagrams
- Is edited and written by leading UK trauma authorities for everyday use by emergency medicine staff, nurses, hospital doctors, paramedics, and ambulance services

DECEMBER 2012 | 9780727918598 | 224 PAGES | £29.99/US$47.95/€38.90/AU$57.95

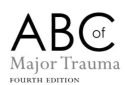
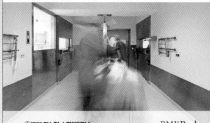

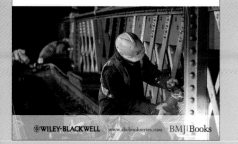

# ABC of Occupational and Environmental Medicine

## 3RD EDITION

**David Snashall & Dipti Patel**

Guy's & St. Thomas' Hospital, London; Medical Advisory Service for Travellers Abroad (MASTA)

Since the publication of last edition, there have been huge changes in the world of occupational health. It has become firmly a part of international public health, and in Britain there is now a National Director for Work and Health. This fully updated new edition embraces these changes and:

- Provides comprehensive guidance on current occupational and environmental health practice and legislation
- Concentrates on the newer kinds of occupational disease, for example 'RSI', pesticide poisoning and electromagnetic radiation, where exposure and effects are difficult to understand
- Places an emphasis on work, health and well-being, and the public health benefits of work, the value of work, disabled people at work, the aging workforce, and vocational rehabilitation
- Includes chapters on the health effects of climate change and of occupational health and safety in relation to migration and terrorism

NOVEMBER 2012 | 9781444338171 | 168 PAGES | £27.99/US$44.95/€38.90/AU$52.95

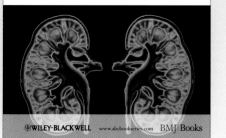

# ABC of Kidney Disease

## 2ND EDITION

**David Goldsmith, Satish Jayawardene & Penny Ackland**

Guy's & St. Thomas' Hospital, London; King's College Hospital, London; Melbourne Grove Medical Practice, London

Nephrology is sometimes considered a complicated and specialized topic and the illustrative ABC format will help GPs quickly and easily assimilate the information needed. *ABC of Kidney Disease, 2nd Edition*:

- Is a practical guide to the most common renal diseases to enable non-renal health care workers to screen, identify, treat and refer renal patients appropriately and to provide the best possible care
- Covers organizational aspects of renal disease management, dialysis and transplantation
- Provides an explanatory glossary of renal terms, guidance on anaemia management and information on drug prescribing and interactions
- Has been fully revised in accordance with new guidelines

OCTOBER 2012 | 9780470672044 | 112 PAGES | £27.99/US$44.95/€35.90/AU$52.95